This book is due for return on or before the last date shown below.

58

31. MAR. 19

Don Gresswell Ltd., London, N.21 Cat. No. 1208

DG 02242/71

ENTERED

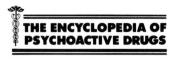

THE ENCYCLOPEDIA OF PSYCHOACTIVE DRUGS

IN 25 VOLUMES
Each title on a specific drug or drug-related problem

CAFFEINE

THE ENCYCLOPEDIA OF PSYCHOACTIVE DRUGS

CAFFEINE

The Most Popular Stimulant

RICHARD J. GILBERT Ph.D.
Addiction Research Foundation of Ontario

GENERAL EDITOR (U.S.A.)
Professor Solomon H. Snyder, M.D.
*Distinguished Service Professor of Neuroscience, Pharmacology
and Psychiatry at
The Johns Hopkins University School of Medicine*

GENERAL EDITOR (U.K.)
Professor Malcolm H. Lader, D.Sc., Ph.D., M.D., F.R.C. Psych.
*Professor of Clinical Psychopharmacology
at the Institute of Psychiatry, University of London,
and Honorary Consultant to the Bethlem Royal and Maudsley
Hospitals*

Burke Publishing Company Limited

LONDON   TORONTO   NEW YORK

Acknowledgements

Photos by courtesy of AP/Wide World Photos, The Bettmann Archive, Dover
Publishers, General Foods Limited, Mary Evans Picture Library, The Photo Co-op,
Sandoz Pharmaceuticals, Weatherhill Publishers.

CIP data

Gilbert, Richard.
   Caffeine – (Encyclopedia of psychoactive drugs)
    1. Caffeine habit   2. Caffeine – Physiological effect
I. Title. II. Series
615'.785 RC567.5
ISBN 0 222 01213 7 Hardbound
ISBN 0 222 01214 5 Paperback

Burke Publishing Company Limited
Pegasus House, 116-120 Golden Lane, London EC1Y 0TL, England.
Printed in Spain by Jerez Industrial S.A.

CONTENTS

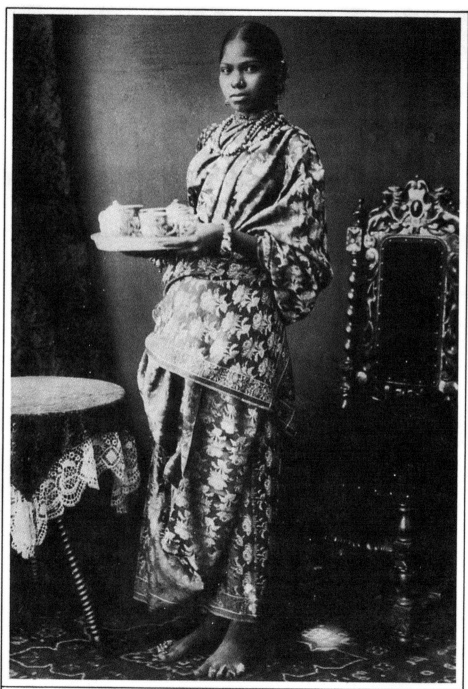

An Indian woman dressed in traditional clothing serves a pot of tea. Tea was first used in Asia as early as 4,700 years ago both as a social drink and for medicinal purposes.

INTRODUCTION

The late twentieth century has seen the rapid growth of both the legitimate medical use and the illicit, non-medical abuse of an increasing number of drugs which affect the mind. Both use and abuse are very high in general in the United States of America and great concern is voiced there. Other Western countries are not far behind and cannot afford to ignore the matter or to shrug off the consequent problems. Nevertheless, differences between countries may be marked and significant: they reflect such factors as social habits, economic status, attitude towards the young and towards drugs and the ways in which health care is provided and laws are enacted and enforced.

Drug abuse particulary concerns the young but other age groups are not immune. Alcoholism in middle-aged men and increasingly in middle-aged women is one example, tranquillizers in women another. Even the old may become alcoholic or dependent on their barbiturates. And the most widespread form of addiction, and the one with the most dire consequences to health, is cigarette-smoking.

Why do so many drug problems start in the teenage and even pre-teenage years? These years are critical in the human life-cycle as they involve maturation from child to adult. During these relatively few years, adolescents face the difficult task of equipping themselves physically and intellectually for adulthood and of establishing goals that make adult life worthwhile while coping with the search for personal identity, assuming their sexual roles and learning to come to terms with authority. During this intense period of growth

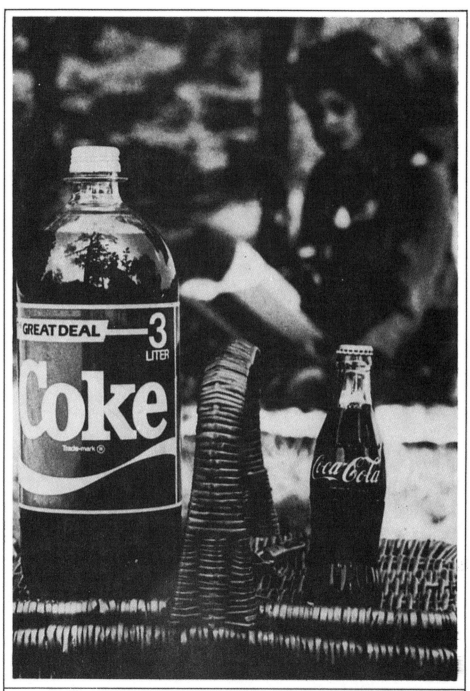

The world's best-selling soft drinks company has recently issued a caffeine-free version of coca-cola. Despite this development, soft drinks are the third largest source of caffeine.

and activity, bewilderment and conflict are inevitable, and peer pressure to experiment and to escape from life's apparent problems becomes overwhelming. Drugs are increasingly available and offer a tempting respite.

Unfortunately, the consequences may be serious. But the penalties for drug-taking must be put into perspective. Thus, addicts die from heroin addiction but people also die from alcoholism and even more from smoking-related diseases. Also, one must separate the direct effects of drug-taking from those indirectly related to the life-style of so many addicts. The problems of most addicts include many factors other than drug-taking itself. The chaotic existence or social deterioration of some may be the cause rather than the effect of drug abuse.

Drug use and abuse must be set into its social context. It reflects a complex interaction between the drug substance (naturally-occurring or synthetic), the person (psychologically normal or abnormal), and society (vigorous or sick). Fads affect drug-taking, as with most other human activities, with drugs being heavily abused one year and unfashionable the next. Such swings also typify society's response to drug abuse. Opiates were readily available in European pharmacies in the last century but are stringently controlled now. Marijuana is accepted and alcohol forbidden in many Islamic countries; the reverse obtains in most Western countries.

The use of psychoactive drugs dates back to prehistory. Opium was used in Ancient Egypt to alleviate pain and its main constituent, morphine, remains a favoured drug for pain relief. Alcohol was incorporated into religious ceremonies in the cradles of civilization in the Near and Middle East and has been a focus of social activity ever since. Coca leaf has been chewed by the Andean Indians to lessen fatigue; and its modern derivative, cocaine, was used as a local anaesthetic. More recently, a succession of psychoactive drugs have been synthesized, developed and introduced into medicine to allay psychological distress and to treat psychiatric illness. But, even so, these innovations may present unexpected problems, such as the difficulties in stopping the long-term use of tranquillizers or slimming-pills, even when taken under medical supervision.

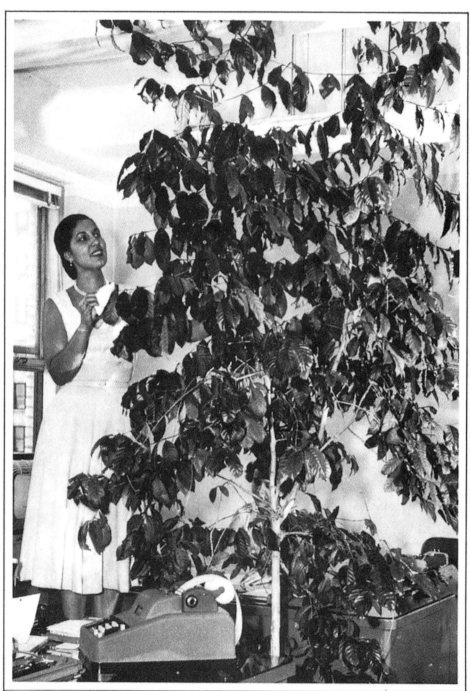

A woman tends a bean-laden coffee plant in her office. Because some coffee plants grow well in air-conditioned places, they have become quite popular office decorations in some countries.

The Encyclopedia of Psychoactive Drugs provides information about the nature of the effects on mind and body of alcohol and drugs and the possible results of abuse. Topics include where the drugs come from, how they are made, how they affect the body and how the body deals with these chemicals; the effects on the mind, thinking, emotions, the will and the intellect are detailed; the processes of use and abuse are discussed, as are the consequences for everyday activities such as school work, employment, driving and dealing with other people. Pointers to identifying drug users and to ways of helping them are provided. In particular, this series aims to dispel myths about drug-taking and to present the facts as objectively as possible without all the emotional distortion and obscurity which surrounds the subject. We seek neither to exaggerate nor to play down the complex topics concerning various forms of drug abuse. We hope that young people will find answers to their questions and that others—parents and teachers, for example—will also find the series helpful.

The series was originally written for American readers by American experts. Often the problem with a drug is particularly pressing in the USA or even largely confined to that country. We have invited a series of British experts to adapt the series for use in non-American English-speaking countries and believe that this widening of scope has successfully increased the relevance of these books to take account of the international drug scene.

In this volume, originally written by Richard J. Gilbert and adapted by Malcolm S. Bruce, the most popular drug in the world, caffeine, is assessed. Used widely as an innocuous "pick-me-up", there are, nevertheless, hazards associated with its use. Direct effects of too much caffeine include anxiety, tension and insomnia. Mild dependence is common so that attempting to cut down or stop the regular use of caffeine-containing beverages may be followed by sleepiness or headache.

Caffeine raises interesting questions concerning the social implications of the medical harm following the use of a widely accepted substance. This book provides the factual basis which the reader can consider in deciding whether to modify his own caffeine intake.

M. H. Lader

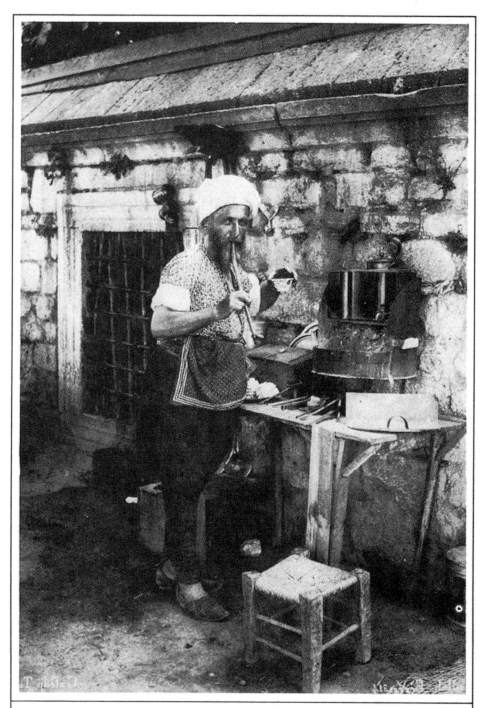

A Turk holds a cup of strong brew made by boiling ground coffee in one of the finjans, *or small, long-handled pots, on the table.*

CHAPTER 1

THE HISTORY OF
TEA AND COFFEE

Caffeine is the most popular drug in the world. Caffeine a drug? Most people recognize two types of drugs. The first type includes chemicals such as aspirin and penicillin that can be purchased at the pharmacy and are used to treat illnesses. And the second type includes substances such as heroin, cocaine, nicotine, and alcohol that people take to relax, to invigorate, or to escape from reality.

Technically, a drug is a chemical substance used to prevent or cure disease or to enhance a person's physical or mental welfare. In fact, people use caffeine for all of these purposes and caffeine can do all of these things, though usually in a very limited way.

Though caffeine is a chemical used both for medical and nonmedical reasons, most often it is used nonmedically for its stimulating effect on mood and behaviour. Drugs that are taken primarily to alter mood or change behaviour are known as *psychoactive drugs.* Heroin, cocaine, marijuana, nicotine, alcohol *and* caffeine are all psychoactive drugs.

Prehistory

Most of the known caffeine-yielding plants were probably discovered and used in paleolithic, or Stone Age times, approximately 600,000 to 700,000 years ago. Paleolithic people chewed the seeds, bark and leaves of many plants and they probably associated the chewing of parts of caffeine-containing plants with the resulting changes in mood and behaviour. Eventually, caffeine was cultivated and consumed to banish fatigue, prolong wakefulness and elevate mood.

Initially, paleolithic people may have ground the caffeine-containing plant material to a paste and used it to aid digestion. Only much later was it discovered that by infusing the plant in hot water, a liquid could be created that when ingested produced greater effects. (This is true because more caffeine is extracted from a plant substance at higher temperatures.) This discovery led to the origin of all the caffeine-containing beverages, including maté, guarana, yoco infusion, cassina, kola tea, coffee, tea and cocoa.

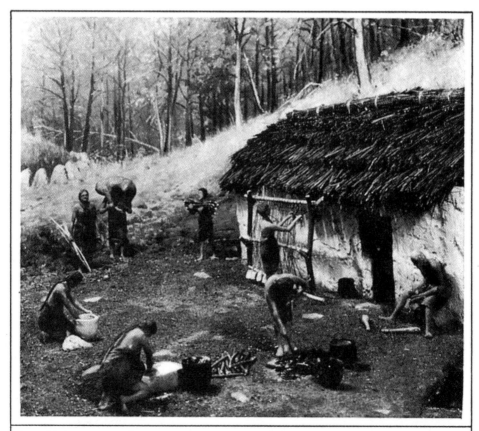

A reconstruction of a Stone Age community at work. Caffeine use has been traced as far back as Paleolithic times, 600,000 years ago.

Tea

Tea has always been used both as a hot beverage and as a medicine. Records indicate that tea drinking may have existed in China as early as 4,700 years ago. Tea use and other aspects of Chinese culture spread to Japan around AD 600, but it took 700 years for it to become fully integrated into Japanese life. In Japan, tea became known by its Cantonese name, *ch'a*. In the 17th century, as the use of coffee was being introduced to Europe from Turkey, Dutch traders brought tea (originally called *tee,* from the Chinese Amoy dialect word *t'e,* pronounced "tay") back to their country. Despite its initial high cost, tea spread quickly throughout Europe and

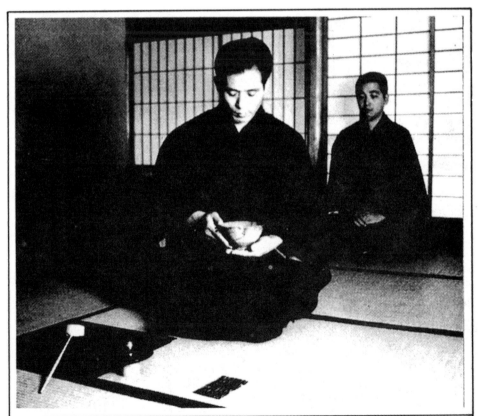

Two men participate in the Japanese tea ceremony, a 600-year-old tradition in which the serving and drinking of tea have become ritualized to create a sacred and aesthetic experience.

in some places displaced coffee as the beverage of choice.

Tea took a particularly strong hold in the North American colonies. American women were "such slaves to it", wrote one tourist in the 1760s, "that they would rather go without their dinners than without a dish of tea".

Partly to reaffirm its status as a strong colonial ruler, in 1767 the British government put a special tax on tea and several other items. As a result, the colonists boycotted tea and began using substitutes, particularly coffee. They were urged on by some local doctors and clergy, who attributed an assortment of ills and evils to tea drinking.

The tea boycott became a rallying point for the growing colonial independence movement. Colonists began destroying cargoes of tea in harbours along the east coast. In Boston on December 16, 1773, a group of citizens disguised as Indians boarded three moored ships and dumped their cargo of tea into the Boston harbour. This incident—the Boston Tea Party—and the British government's reprisals helped precipitate the American Revolution.

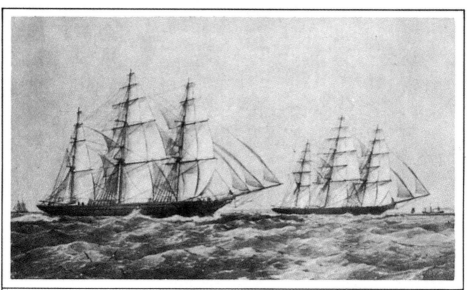

Bearing the season's tea crop for different companies, the clippers Taiping *and* Ariel *race each other from China to Britain in 1866. The tea trade was highly competitive in the 19th century.*

At first, the British did not realize the full significance of the Boston incident. Reports in London newspapers a month later focused not so much on the political implications of the event as on the effect of the tea on the unfortunate fish in the harbour. The fish, said one report, "had contracted a disorder not unlike the nervous complaints of the body". In fact, the large quantity of tea dumped into the harbour had given the fish a strong dose of caffeine.

At this time most tea came from China. Through the East India Company, the British had a near monopoly on the tea trade. When the company's commercial treaty with China expired in 1833, however, the British control of the valuable tea trade became increasingly insecure. During the rest of the 19th century, tea plantations were developed in the Indian

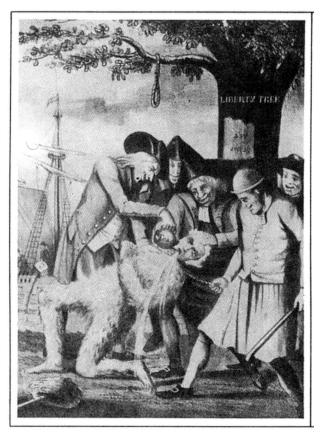

Patriotic colonists tar and feather a tax collector. The demonstration against the imposed tea tariff culminated with the Boston Tea Party on December 16, 1773, when a group of Bostonians, disguised as Indians, boarded a ship owned by the British East India Company and dumped 342 chests of tea into the harbour.

subcontinent. But China tea did not grow well in India, and the plantations became successful only when the local Assam variety of tea was cultivated. As recently as the 1870s more than 90% of Britain's tea still came from China.

The insecurity of Britain's hold on the tea trade was not helped by a domestic tax on tea that, in the early 19th century, was 15 times higher than the tax on coffee. As a consequence, coffee use in Britain increased tenfold between 1800 and 1840, at which time the beverage overtook tea in popularity. A series of coffee-adulteration scandals, however, led many people to return to tea. To the distress of buyers and drinkers, chicory, roasted corn, vegetable roots and baked horse liver were discovered as having been used to increase the bulk of ground coffee. Also, in the mid-nineteenth century, the taxes on tea were lowered. Thus, tea once again became the beverage of choice for the British.

Another country in which tea has been extremely popular is Ireland, although Prime Minister Eamon de Valera attempted to ban the drink in the 1930s. In a symbolic effort to rid his country of British influence, which he claimed was preventing the full flowering of national aspiration, de Valera led the movement to ban tea by promoting indigenous milk and beer as alternatives. The campaign, however, was unsuccessful, and today Ireland remains the leading non-Arabian tea-drinking country in the world.

Coffee

The first written mention of coffee is found in Arabian documents of the 10th century. There is evidence though, that in Ethiopia coffee was cultivated and the berries chewed as early as the 6th century. An Arabian legend tells of a young goatherd who discovered the stimulative effect of the berries after noticing that his goats became very frisky after grazing on coffee bushes. Coffee berries were still being chewed in tropical Africa in the 19th century. Before the Arabian peoples took to making a hot drink from beans, they crushed them, fermented the juice and made a wine called *qahwah*. When at the beginning of the 11th century they began to use the beans to produce the hot drink, they also called it *qahwah*. As use of the drink spread throughout the world this word was adapted to the various languages of coffee-using people, producing such words as cafe, Kaffee, Koffie and coffee.

By the end of the 17th century the Dutch had established coffee plantations on the Indonesian island of Java. During the next 50 years, first the French and then the British followed suit in their Caribbean colonies. Commercial cultivation of coffee spread from the Caribbean to Central and South America, and by the early 19th century Brazil had supplanted Indonesia as the major producer and exporter of coffee. By 1860 the United States was consuming three quarters of the world's coffee, more than half of which came from Brazil.

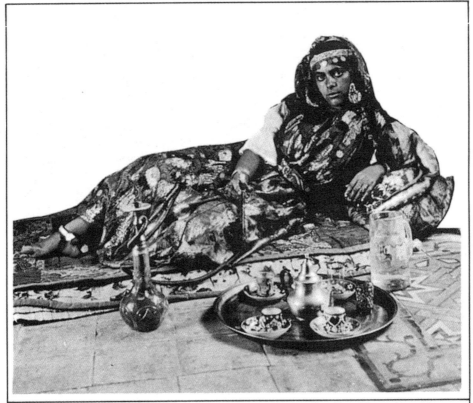

A Moorish woman lounges next to her water pipe and coffee. There is evidence that coffee berries were chewed in Africa as far back as the 6th century, 500 years before the hot drink was first produced.

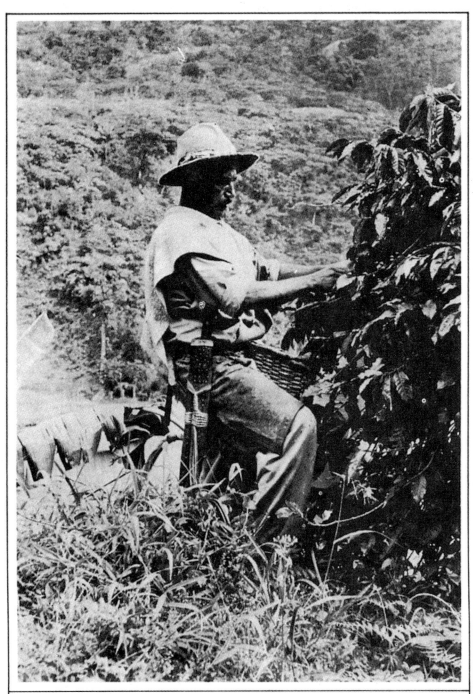

A coffee picker at work in Colombia, berries are picked at optimum grades of ripeness, requiring the picker to return to the same tree several times during harvest and pick the red berries one at a time.

CHAPTER 2

SOURCES OF CAFFEINE

Nearly all of the approximately 120,000 tonnes of caffeine consumed in the world each year comes from coffee and tea plants. About 54% of this caffeine comes from coffee beans and 43% comes from tea leaves. The remaining 3% comes mostly from cacao pods, which are the basis of cocoa butter and chocolate, and also from nuts, maté leaves and many other sources. Only a very small amount of caffeine is chemically synthesized in laboratories.

Not all of the caffeine derived from coffee and tea plants ends up in coffee mugs and tea cups. A considerable amount is extracted from low-quality coffee beans and tea leaves or is collected as a by-product of the decaffeination of coffee and tea. This caffeine is used in soft drinks and in medicines.

The beans used to produce coffee grow on only three species: *Coffea arabica,* native to Ethiopia, is now cultivated chiefly in Brazil and Colombia; *Coffea robusta,* native to Saudi Arabia, is now cultivated chiefly in Indonesia, Brazil and many parts of Africa; and *Coffea liberica,* native to Liberia, is currently cultivated in Africa. Tea leaves used in brewing tea grow on a single species, *Camellia sinensis,* native to China and India where it is still chiefly cultivated. Wild species of both genuses grow abundantly — *Coffea* in Africa and *Camellia* in the Yunnan province of China, where a 1,800-year-old plant over 90 feet tall has been reported.

The other commercially valuable plant sources of caffeine are cocoa beans and kola nuts, produced mainly in

Africa, and maté leaves, guarana seeds and yoco bark, all of which grow in South America. Only maté is consumed in any quantity, and then only in Paraguay, Uruguay and Argentina. Table 1 summarizes the information about these major sources of caffeine. One should note that because tea is made with approximately four times as much water per weight as is coffee, a cup of coffee contains roughly twice as much caffeine as a cup of tea.

Table 1

Sources of Caffeine					
SOURCE	PLANT PART	COUNTRY OF ORIGIN	CURRENT MAIN CULTIVATION SITE	MEANS OF CAFFEINE INTAKE	TYPICAL CAFFEINE CONTENT (% weight)
Coffee bean *Coffea arabica L.* *Coffea robusta* *Coffea liberica*	seed seed seed	Ethiopia Arabia Liberia	Brazil, Colombia Indonesia, Africa Africa	coffee coffee coffee	1.1 2.2 1.4
Tea *Camellia sinensis*	leaf, bud	China	India, China	tea	3.5
Kola nut *Cola acuminata S.* *Cola nitida*	seed	West Africa	West Africa	chewing nuts kola tea	1.5
Cacao pod *Theobroma cacao L.*	seed	Mexico	West Africa, Brazil	cocoa and chocolate products	0.03 1.7
Maté *Ilex paraquayensis*	leaf,	South America	South America	yerba maté	less than 0.7
Yaupon *Ilex cassine* *I. vomitoria*	leaf berry	North America	(not cultivated)	cassina	unknown
Guarana paste *Paullinia capana* *P. sorbilis*	seed	Brazil	Brazil	guarana bars and drink	more than 4
Yoco *Paullinia yoco*	bark	South America	South America	yoco infusion	2.7

SOURCE: G.A. Spiller ed. *The Methylxanthine Beverages & Foods.* New York: Alan R. Liss, 1984.

Why Plants Contain Caffeine

To understand why certain plants have evolved to contain caffeine, researchers have focused on how this chemical compound might benefit these plants. One idea is that caffeine-containing plants gain protection from attack by bacteria, fungi and insects. Caffeine is known to inhibit the actions of bacteria and fungi, and to cause sterility in certain insects, which decreases the insect population. In addition, because caffeine gets into the surrounding soil, it may inhibit the growth of weeds that might otherwise destroy the plants. Obviously, a plant containing a substance that gives it this kind of protection will have a higher survival rate than one that either has a smaller amount or none at all.

However, if caffeine were to harm the plant itself this advantage would be lost. In fact, caffeine-containing plants do have mechanisms for protecting themselves against the caffeine's poisonous effects. For example, coffee plants produce and store the caffeine in coffee seedlings, away from the sites of cell division, which is very sensitive to toxic substances. But caffeine may still eventually kill the coffee

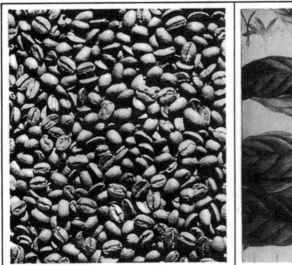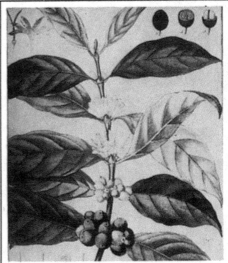

Roasted coffee beans (left) from Coffea arabica, *illustrated here with both ripe and immature berries. Cross-sections of two berries show that each one contains two coffee beans.*

plants that produced it. As a caffeine-bearing bush or tree ages, the soil around it becomes increasingly rich in caffeine that it has absorbed from the accumulation of the plant's fallen leaves and berries. It is partially because of this that coffee plantations tend to degenerate after 10 to 25 years.

Coffee Cultivation

Coffea arabica, which accounts for about 75% of all coffee consumption, is an evergreen tree or shrub that grows best in areas with moderate rainfall and at altitudes of between 2,000 feet (609.6m) and 6,500 feet (1981.2m) above sea level. In Ecuador it is cultivated as high as 9,400 feet (2865m), while in subtropical Hawaii it is grown near the sea. It is also necessary for the temperature to remain as close as possible to 68°F (20°C). The variety that is cultivated commercially grows to a height of approximately 16 feet (4.88m), though to ease harvesting it is frequently trimmed to a height of about 6 feet (1.83m).

Three or four years after planting, *Coffea arabica* produces highly scented blossoms. The coffee berries ripen six to eight months later, changing from dark green to yellow, then to red, and eventually to deep crimson when they are fully ripe. Because of their size and general appearance, the ripe berries are known as coffee cherries. Beneath the

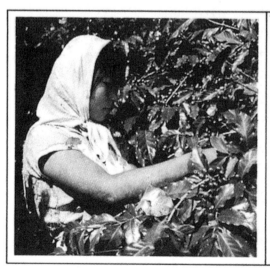

A woman picking coffee berries in Brazil. Because a tree can bear ripe and unripe berries at the same time, the ripe berries must be singled out and then picked by hand. A worker must pick 2,000 berries in order to produce a single pound of roasted coffee.

crimson skin of the cherry is a moist, soft, sweet-tasting pulp that surrounds the green coffee bean. The bean itself has a thin, delicate, translucent covering known as the silver skin.

The proper time to harvest varies according to climate and altitude. Where conditions are less than ideal, as in southern Brazil, coffee is harvested only in the winter. Under perfect conditions, as in Java, planting is staggered throughout the year, and therefore the coffee can be harvested almost continuously. The berries are picked by hand or shaken from the bush onto mats.

Coffea arabica is a delicate plant which is plagued by more than 40 diseases caused by fungi, viruses, bacteria and soil deficiencies. The worst disease is leaf rust caused by the fungus *Hemileia vastatrix.* The leaves die and drop off, and after a few years the bush dies. Leaf rust damage is a problem almost everywhere except in Central and South America, where farmers destroy the plants at the first sign of the disease. The farmers' success in fighting leaf rust there is why this is where most Arabica coffee is grown. Other, less serious diseases do occur, but mostly where growing conditions are marginal.

Coffea robusta (also known as *Coffea canephora* var. *robusta*) is grown mostly outside the Americas, although some is grown in Brazil. It is more tolerant of extremes of soil and climate and more resistant to diseases and insects than is *Coffea arabica. Coffea robusta* will also grow at lower altitudes. *C. robusta* berries take from two to three months longer to ripen than do *C. arabica* berries, though they typically yield larger harvests. In addition, harvesting is easier because the *C. robusta* berries stay on the tree when they are overripe. These differences mean that it costs less to grow *C. robusta* coffee, and this cost difference accounts for the increasing use of this coffee plant, despite its reportedly inferior taste.

Coffee Processing

There are two methods used to separate the bean from the berry. In the *wet process,* a pulping machine breaks open the freshly picked berries and removes the skin and some of the flesh beneath. They are then left in water for about 24 hours, during which time more of the flesh is loosened by the action of yeasts and bacteria (fermentation). Afterwards, the beans are washed and then dried in the sun. Finally their silver skin is removed and they are machine polished. This yields what are known by coffee traders as *green beans.* This wet process, used for all Arabica coffee berries except for those in Brazil, generally produces a higher grade of bean.

Dry processing is a less expensive method of separating the bean from the berry and is used for almost all Robusta coffees and for Arabica coffees in Brazil. In this method the berries are stripped from the plant and either dried in special machines or left to dry in the sun for two to three weeks. After this period the dried husks and silver skins are readily removed by machinery or even by hand to yield the green coffee beans. Dry processing produces beans which create a harsher tasting coffee than those beans processed by the wet method. For this reason Arabica coffee from Brazil tends not to be of the highest quality. When *C. robusta* berries are wet processed, as they are in Uganda, the result is a bean that is better than most other Robustas.

Under the right conditions, green coffee beans may be

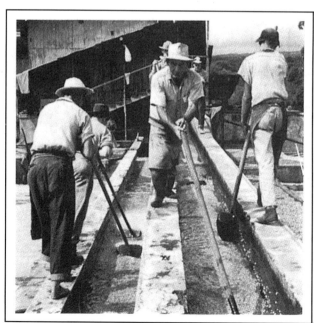

The wet process converts the coffee berry to ready-for-export green coffee beans. The beans, which have been depulped by machine, travel by sluiceway to the drying area. In these sluiceways, fresh water removes any substances that may be clinging to the beans.

stored for many years. They are usually exported in 60-kg (132.276 lbs) bags, although there is a growing international trade in processed (soluble or instant) coffee.

Much of the coffee that is consumed undergoes further processing to produce decaffeinated coffee. Because some of the oils and other flavour components of the coffee bean are lost during the various processes, the stronger tasting Robustas and the dry-processed Arabicas from Brazil are generally used.

In an attempt to remove 97% or more of the caffeine, while leaving or returning to the bean as much of the flavour components as possible, manufacturers use many techniques. If the *direct-contact method* is used, the green coffee beans are first steamed until they are hot, wet and swollen. Then the caffeine is extracted using a chemical solvent, such as methylene chloride. (Trichlorethylene was widely used until the mid-1970s, when it was found that high doses caused liver cancer in mice.) Finally the beans are steamed to wash away the solvent.

The *water extraction method,* popular in Europe though more expensive than the direct contact method, produces a

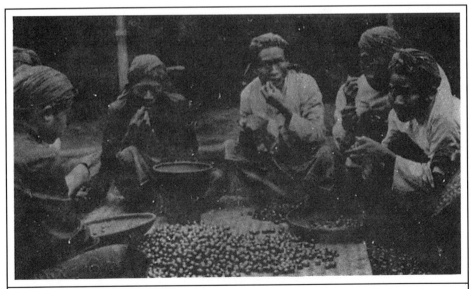

Indonesian workers, displaying a type of dry processing, crack the coffee berry open with their teeth in order to remove the coffee beans.

better tasting drink. In this process, hot water is recycled continuously through the green beans until 97% of the caffeine is removed. Then a solvent is used to extract the caffeine from the water, which is used again to extract caffeine from a new batch of beans. Because this water already contains coffee-flavour components, a lesser amount of them are extracted from subsequent batches, and therefore the beans retain much of their original flavour.

Roasting of both regular and decaffeinated green beans is generally carried out shortly before it reaches the retail market. This is done commercially by passing the green beans through 260°C (500°F) gases for up to 5 minutes, the length of roasting time depending on the desired darkness of the bean which in turn affects the taste and caffeine content of the brewed coffee. The bean loses water during roasting— 14% during the shortest roast, known as "light city", which produces a cinnamon-coloured bean, and 20% during the longest roast, known as "Italian", which produces a dark brown to black bean. The final step before brewing is grinding, which is usually done by the processor or in the store, but increasingly it is being done at the point of preparation in homes or restaurants so that no flavour is lost.

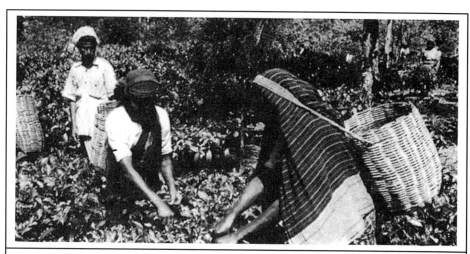

Women harvesting tea in India. A worker can pick about 3,000 shoots of tea a day, which produces less than one pound of manufactured tea.

Instant coffee is produced from the roasted beans using one of two methods. Both begin by brewing a coffee extract in huge percolators. Pressurized water at 135°C (338°F) is used to force more of the bean into solution. In the manufacture of *spray-dried coffee* the extract is fed into the top of a tower of hot air. This dries the extract into a powder, which can be recovered from the bottom of the tower. *Freeze-dried coffee,* more expensive though better tasting, takes advantage of the fact that the water and the solids in the coffee extract separate upon freezing. Afterwards the solids are granulated or turned into flakes.

Tea Cultivation

The tea plant, *Camellia sinensis,* has a great number of varieties, or subspecies. Considerable confusion once existed as to whether there was one or more species of the plant, but in 1958 it was internationally agreed that there is one species with several varieties, of which two have major commercial importance.

Like the coffee plant, the tea plant is an evergreen tree or bush that grows in the tropics or subtropics. It grows best at altitudes of between 2,000 (609.6m) and 6,500 feet

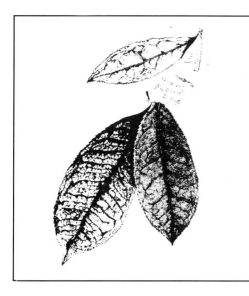

All types of tea come from the same species of plant, Camellia sinensis *(above). Differences in local climate, cultivating conditions and methods of manufacture account for the fact that there are over 2,000 different blends of tea.*

31

(1981.2m) and in areas that receive moderate rainfall. The most cultivated variety is Assam tea, or var. *assamica,* which because of its low resistance to cold survives best in tropical areas. China tea, or var. *sinensis,* has lower yields than Assam tea but produces a more delicately flavoured beverage. It can tolerate brief cold periods and thus higher altitudes than Assam tea. In the late 1800s China tea was cultivated in South Carolina, but the plantations were abandoned because high labour costs made them economically unsound. However, many plants still survive in this area.

The Assam tea plant has large leaves, up to 10 inches (25.4cm) long, and if left uncultivated can grow to a height of 50 feet (15.24m). The China tea plant is smaller, with 4-inch (10.16cm) leaves and a natural height of no more than 20 feet (6.096m). Both plants are trimmed to waist height to facilitate plucking of the leaves. Ideally, only young leaves and shoots are harvested. Plucking only the young leaves in such a way as to keep the plant healthy is a highly skilled job. Though to reduce labour costs mechanical shearing is on the increase; this method produces a coarse tea of varying quality.

Tea Processing

After plucking, the leaves are most frequently treated in one of two ways. About three-quarters of the leaves are made into *black tea;* the other quarter becomes *green tea,* the type generally drunk in China and often served in Chinese restaurants. Because of the type of equipment required, the manufacture of black tea is carried out almost exclusively in large factories. Green tea can be produced under the small-scale conditions of the family farm, though today it is most frequently manufactured on a larger scale. To produce black tea, freshly plucked leaves are withered and then squeezed or minced to release their sap. The sap contains the enzyme (an organic catalyst) *tea polyphenol oxidase,* which causes the plant's colourless flavour-producing chemicals to take up oxygen from the air. This oxidizing process changes the leaves' character and in addition turns them dark brown.

To produce green tea, the oxidizing enzyme is destroyed before it can cause changes in colour and flavour. This is done by heat—steam heat in Japan and dry heat in China.

Because it contains unoxidized flavour-producing substances, green tea tends to have a more bitter flavour than black tea. After this initial step is completed, the leaves are treated much as black tea. Both teas contain a similar amount of caffeine.

After manufacture, the tea is sorted by size, purged of stalks and dust, packed in foil-lined chests and shipped to blenders or auctioneers. Each chest contains between 30 kg (66.138lbs) and 60 kg (132.276lbs) of tea leaf. In North America, more than 90% of tea is packaged in the form of tea bags.

A small portion of the tea is further processed to remove the caffeine or to produce instant tea. The decaffeination of tea is very similar to the decaffeination of coffee, most often utilizing the same solvent, methylene chloride, to extract the caffeine from the moistened leaf.

Instant tea, unpopular in the UK since most is used to make iced tea, is also manufactured in a manner similar to that of instant coffee. Firstly, an extract is prepared by subjecting the leaves to high temperature and high pressure water. Then the extract is spray-dried to produce a powder. Further processing may be required to ensure that the powder is soluble in cold water. Prior to marketing, the tea powder is often blended with a sweetener and/or lemon flavouring.

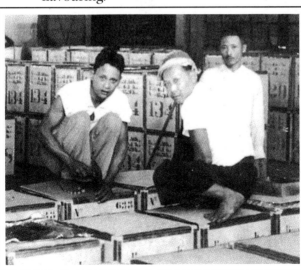

Workers in a Southeast Asian country pack tea in foil-lined boxes prior to shipping in order to preserve flavour.

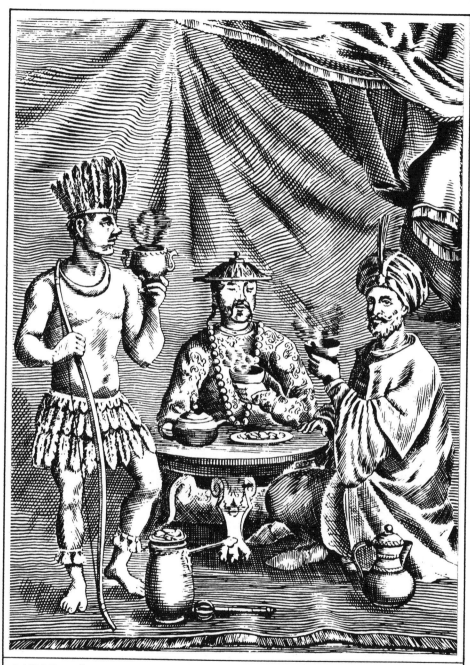

A 1688 French engraving, "Treatises on Coffee, Tea and Chocolate". By weight tea leaves have more than twice as much caffeine as coffee beans, but a cup of coffee has twice as much of the drug because more beans are used in the brew. Though cocoa has a much lower amount of caffeine, it contains large amounts of the stimulant theobromine.

CHAPTER 3

CAFFEINE'S CHEMISTRY AND BIOCHEMISTRY

Pure caffeine is a bitter-tasting white powder that resembles cornstarch. It is moderately soluble in water at body temperature and readily soluble in boiling water. It was first isolated from coffee in 1820 and from tea in 1827 and given the name *theine.* Soon thereafter it was recognized that the mood- and behaviour-altering properties of both coffee and tea depended upon caffeine.

Caffeine has two technical names. The full name is 3,7-dihydro-1,3,7-trimethyl-1 H-purine-2,6-dione. The more commonly used technical name is 1,3,7-trimethylxanthine. Both names describe the chemical structure of the caffeine molecule, whose two-dimensional representation is shown in Figure 1. Its chemical formula is $C_8H_{10}N_4O_2$.

To understand caffeine's effects, a brief introduction to purine and its related compounds is necessary (see Figure 1). Purine is the parent compound of all of these chemicals and of many other of the important chemicals found in the body. Upon closer inspection it can be seen that xanthine, or *dioxypurine,* is purine with two oxygen atoms, and that caffeine, or *trimethylxanthine,* is xanthine with three methyl groups. As shown, a methyl group consists of a carbon atom and three hydrogen atoms. The "1,3,7" in caffeine's technical names refers to the positions of the methyl groups, as numbered in the purine structure.

Purine does not occur in the body in its pure form. When chemicals in the purine family are broken down, xanthine is produced as an intermediate product. The liver further converts xanthine into uric acid, which is found in unusually high levels in humans. Though too much uric acid is associated with the disease known as gout, uric acid is believed to contribute to our living longer than most other mammals.

The two most important purines found in the body are adenine and guanine. These two, together with cytosine and thymine, comprise the four basic letters of the genetic alphabet, or code, found in the cells of all living organisms. Everything a person inherits—from membership in the human species to eye colour—is determined by this code. The code is "read" in groups of three purines, each chemically bound to a long strand of molecules. Two strands and their purines make up what is called a DNA, or deoxyribonucleic acid, double helix. Genes are sequences of the groups of three purines found at specific places on the chromosomes, structures composed of DNA (see Figure 2).

The duplication of DNA is one of the central processes in the reproduction of cells and whole organisms. Caffeine,

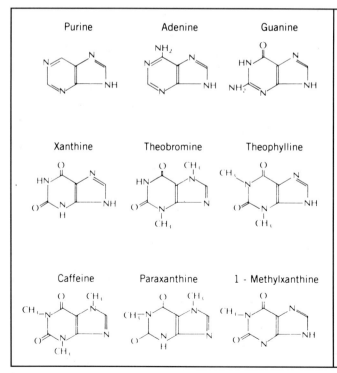

Figure 1. *A chart of different chemical compounds with similar structures: purine, the parent compound; adenine and guanine, two of the four compounds that form the genetic code; xanthine, a product of the breakdown of purines in the body; the dimethylxanthines theobromine and theophylline; caffeine, a trimethylxanthine, or xanthine with three methyl groups; paraxanthine and 1-methylxanthine, metabolites of caffeine.*

because of its similarity to critical parts of the genetic code, can interfere with this process and cause errors in the cells' reproduction. This may result in tumours, cancers and genetic defects. The significance of caffeine's effects on reproduction is discussed further in Chapter 12.

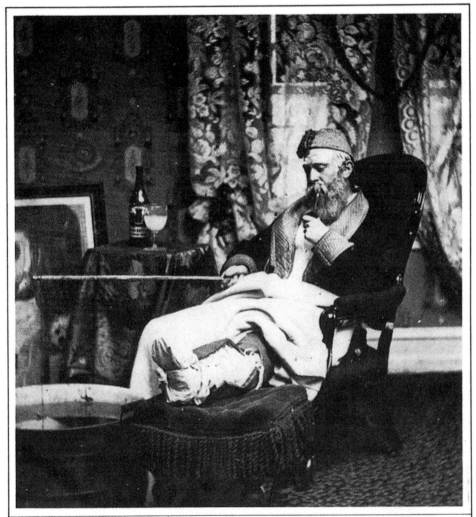

A person suffering from gout, a disease marked by painful swelling of the joints. Gout is caused by a high level of uric acid in the body, produced during the liver's breakdown of purines such as caffeine.

Theobromine and Theophylline

Theobromine and theophylline are two dimethylxanthines, or xanthine molecules that have two rather than three methyl groups (see Figure 1). Both dimethylxanthines produce effects similar to caffeine's, though their relative potencies are different. Approximately equivalent stimulating effects would be given by, 10mg theophylline, 50mg caffeine, and 200mg theobromine.

Theobromine is found in cocoa products, tea (only in very small amounts) and kola nuts, but is not found in coffee. In cocoa, theobromine's concentration is generally about seven times as great as caffeine's. Because of this, although the caffeine content of cocoa products is relatively low, the actual caffeine-like effects produced by consuming these products will still be significant.

Theophylline, found in very small amounts with caffeine and theobromine in tea, has a stronger stimulatory effect than caffeine on the heart and on breathing. It is often the drug of choice in treating diseases in which breathing is difficult, such as asthma, bronchitis, and emphysema. The theophylline used in medicine is made from caffeine extracted from coffee or tea.

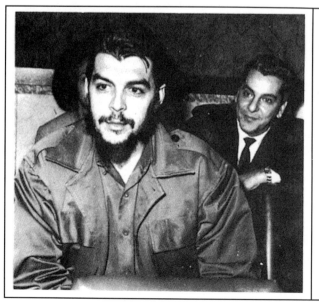

Ernesto "Che" Guevara, a well-known revolutionary leader, drank yerba maté, a caffeine-rich drink popular in Latin America, to ease his asthma.

The Body's Absorption of Caffeine

Caffeine is moderately soluble in water and therefore can be found in the body wherever there is water—which is in most places. Caffeine also readily passes through cell membranes. Because of these properties, after caffeine is ingested it is rapidly and completely absorbed from the stomach and intestines into the bloodstream, which distributes it to all organs of the body, including the brain, the ovaries and the testes. In addition, when a pregnant woman consumes a caffeine-containing food, the drug quickly goes to all of the organs of the unborn child.

In the bloodstream caffeine finally travels to the liver, where, by a process known as *metabolism,* it is converted into a number of breakdown products known as *metabolites,* which are eventually excreted in the urine. These metabolites include both theobromine, theophylline and a third dimethylxanthine, known as paraxanthine (see Figure 1).

Relatively high levels of paraxanthine are found in the

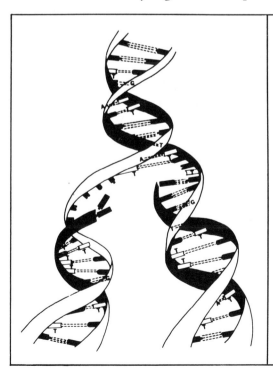

Figure 2. *An illustration of the DNA molecule. Because caffeine is similar in structure to adenine and guanine, two critical parts of the genetic code, it can interfere with the duplication of DNA and cause mutations, or errors, in cell reproduction, which can result in genetic defects.*

blood after caffeine has been ingested. However, as the blood passes through the liver again, paraxanthine is itself broken down to 1-methylxanthine (see Figure 1). Methylxanthine is the main metabolite of caffeine found in human urine, but typically it accounts for only about one-fifth of the caffeine dose. The remainder is turned into one of at least a dozen other products of caffeine metabolism.

Because caffeine so readily passes in both directions across membranes, it is not easily excreted by the kidneys into urine. If caffeine were not metabolized to compounds such as 1-methylxanthine that do not pass back across the kidney membrane and into the bloodstream, the caffeine from a cup of coffee would stay in the body for several days.

Frequently the metabolites of a drug have more effect than the drug that was originally ingested. Paraxanthine and, especially, 1-methylxanthine, are even more similar to adenine and guanine than caffeine itself. Though it is not yet known exactly how much caffeine's metabolites contribute to caffeine's effects, both paraxanthine and 1-methylxanthine may very well play an important part in this drug's stimulation of the nervous system.

Caffeine's Effects

Caffeine's stimulatory effects involve the action of adenosine, a chemical widespread in the body (see Figure 3). The

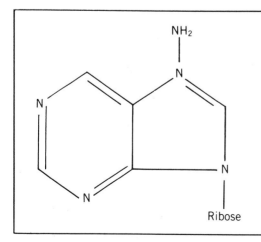

NH₂

Ribose

Figure 3. *The chemical adenosine (left) binds to receptor sites on the cell surface and thus inhibits the release of neurotransmitters, which causes sleepiness. Because of caffeine's structural similarity to adenosine, it can block adenosine's effects by binding to the receptor sites first and stimulating the neurotransmitters.*

adenosine molecule, composed of a purine linked to a type of sugar, is part of a larger molecule that supplies energy necessary for all cell functions.

Adenosine is also an important regulator of body processes, particularly the transmission of signals by nerves. Injection of adenosine or substances that increase adenosine levels can cause lethargy and sleep. Adenosine can also dilate blood vessels, diminish gastrointestinal motility (the gastro-intestinal organs' ability to contract), protect against seizures, retard the body's reaction to stress, and lower heart rate, blood pressure and body temperature.

Adenosine inhibits the release of neurotransmitters, or chemicals that carry messages from one nerve cell to another. To do this it must first bind to specific receptor sites on the cell surface. Because its structure is so similar to adenosine's, caffeine also binds to the receptors, and, in doing so, caffeine prevents adenosine from binding there. Thus, the nerve cells fire more rapidly. Researchers have discovered that both paraxanthine and 1-methylxanthine are even more effective than caffeine in competing with adenosine for adenosine receptors. Therefore, caffeine's brain-stimulating effects may be enhanced by its being metabolized to paraxanthine and 1-methylxanthine.

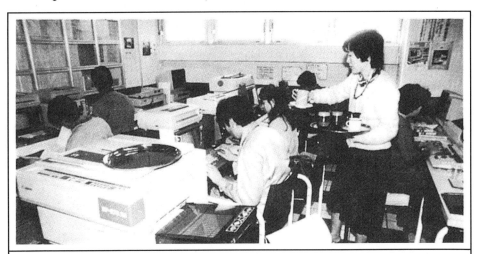

In this "word processing coffeeshop" in Tokyo, customers are served coffee while working at the computers.

41

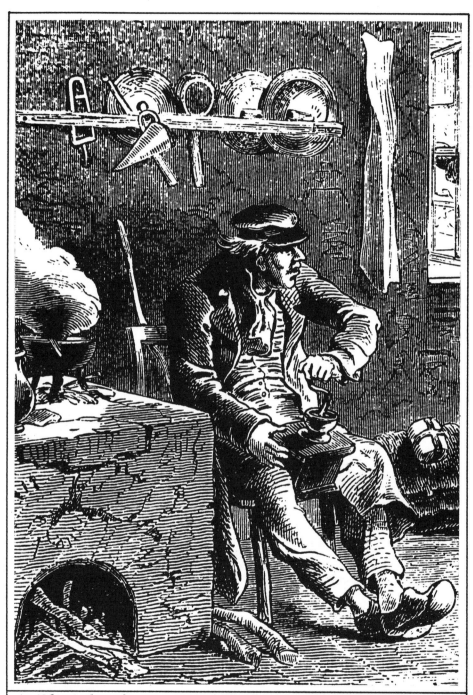

An 1864 woodcut of a man using a box coffee grinder prior to brewing. Coffee is usually ground by the manufacturer, but many households prefer to grind the beans themselves in order to preserve flavour.

CHAPTER 4

HOW CAFFEINE IS USED

*T*he amount of caffeine in cups of coffee and tea varies enormously (see Table 2). Excluding decaffeinated coffees and teas, the range for coffee is from 29 to 176 mg and the range for tea is from 8 to 91 mg. This wide variance is mainly due to the size of the cup and the quantity and quality of the coffee bean or tea leaf used. Because of this it can be very difficult to compare two people's intake by simply asking them how many cups of coffee or cups of tea they drink.

Drip coffee contains more caffeine than percolated coffee, which in turn contains more caffeine than instant coffee. The large difference in caffeine content between drip and percolated coffee found in home-prepared drinks is probably an indication that more coffee bean per cup was used to make drip coffee. In making drip coffee the water passes over the ground bean only once, while in a percolator it repeatedly passes over the ground bean. In fact, nearly all of the caffeine is dissolved in the near-boiling water during the first pass, especially if the bean is ground finely. Repeated

Table 2

Caffeine Content of Standard Drink Servings	
Average cup of coffee	80 milligrams
Strong cup of coffee	120 milligrams
Average cup of tea	40 milligrams
Average can or bottle of caffeine-containing soft drink	40 milligrams

SOURCE: Gilbert, R.M., et al., *Canadian Medical Association Journal,* and Blanch, J.L., *Journal of Food Science.*

passing only causes more of the other coffee bean components to go into solution. These other components add to the
bitterness of the drink, and thus its apparent strength, though
the caffeine content is only very minimally affected. To
decrease the bitterness, people tend to use less bean when
percolating coffee.

The variation in the caffeine content of home-prepared
cups of tea is even greater than that for coffee. The variables
here are the amount of tea leaf used (or the size of the tea
bag), cup size, and the time the tea is left to brew. Caffeine is
released from tea leaves a little more slowly than from coffee
beans, especially if the leaves are in tea bags.

Caffeine is a constituent not only of cups of coffee and
tea, including iced tea, but also of foods and drinks that are
flavoured with coffee or tea.

Caffeine in Soft Drinks

In hot countries, the next most important source of caffeine,
after tea and coffee is soft drinks (see Table 3). In 1982
between 65 and 86% of the soft drinks sold in the United
States contained caffeine. During the following two years,
aggressive marketing of caffeine-free soft drinks reduced that
percentage. Figures suggest that by the end of 1983 a wholly
new brand, Diet Coke, had moved ahead of all other brands as
the leading seller among caffeine-free soft drinks.

More than 95% of the caffeine in soft drinks is added

Table 3

Market Share and Caffeine Content of Popular Caffeine-Containing Soft Drinks in USA		
BRAND	MARKET SHARE IN 1982	CAFFEINE CONTENT (mg/12oz)
Coca-Cola*	23.9%	46
Pepsi-Cola*	18.1%	38
Dr Pepper*	5.1%	40
Tab	3.8%	47
Mountain Dew*	2.8%	54

*Diet versions of these brands contain the same or almost the same amounts of caffeine.

SOURCE: Soft Drink Manufacturers Association

during manufacture. The remainder comes from the kola nut, the ingredient for which cola drinks were named when they were first introduced in the 1880s. At that time, Coca-Cola, the first of the colas, also contained cocaine, which occurs naturally in coca leaves. Since 1903 the coca leaves used in the manufacture of colas have been decocainized, although manufacturers have not been required to demonstrate the absence of cocaine since 1969. Today, Coke probably contains very small amounts of cocaine.

Caffeine in Cocoa and Chocolate

Cocoa and chocolate products are the next most important sources of caffeine (see Table 4). The range of caffeine content in these products varies considerably, although the caffeine content of these products is relatively low. Only chocolate bars contain a significant amount of caffeine, and here the range is also great. Only the finest quality sweet, or

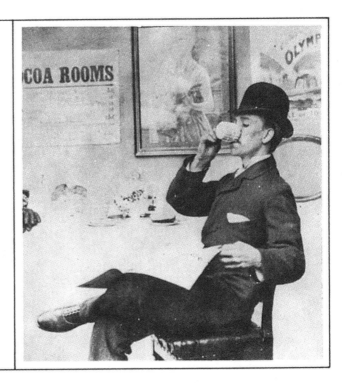

Cocoa bars were popular around 1900. Cocoa was introduced to the European countries in 1528, nearly a century before coffee and tea, but its use spread very slowly. Eventually, however, chocolate houses such as this one became fashionable.

dark chocolate has a high caffeine content. The typical 50-gram milk chocolate bar sold has about 10 mg of caffeine if it is mostly chocolate, and much less if there is a substantial quantity of nonchocolate filler such as nuts and fudge, or if some or all of the chocolate is artificial.

The theobromine content of each item is also given in Table 4. As previously mentioned, theobromine is similar to caffeine in structure and effect on the body, though it is only one-quarter as potent. However, cocoa and chocolate products typically have approximately 10 times as much theobromine as caffeine. Therefore, the caffeine-like effects produced by consuming a cocoa or chocolate product will be greater than one might expect from the actual caffeine content.

Caffeine in Medicines

The final important source of caffeine is prescription and over-the-counter drugs. All of this caffeine is also added during manufacture. Table 5 gives the caffeine content per tablet or capsule of some commonly used drugs. Why caffeine should be a component of these drugs is discussed in depth in Chapter 10.

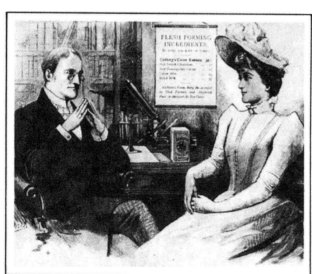

Some women in the late 19th century worried that they were too thin. To help them gain weight, doctors sometimes recommended products such as Cadbury's Cocoa Essence, which contained cocoa as one of its "flesh-forming ingredients".

Table 4

Caffeine and Theobromine Content of Cocoa and Chocolate Products			
PRODUCT	SERVING SIZE	CAFFEINE (mg)	THEOBROMINE (mg)
Chocolate bar	50 grams	3–63	68–314
Hot cocoa	150 millilitres	1–8	40–80
Chocolate Milk	225 millilitres	2–7	35–99
Chocolate ice cream	50 grams	2–5	15–39

SOURCE: G.A. Spiller, ed. *The Methylxanthine Beverages & Foods.* New York: Alan R. Liss, 1984.

Table 5

Caffeine Content of Some Common Drug Preparations	
CLASSIFICATION	AMOUNT PER TABLET OR CAPSULE (mg)
OVER-THE-COUNTER DRUGS	
Analgesics	
Anadin	15
Beechams tab	25
Hedex plus	30
Anadin Extra	45
Beechams Powders	50
Phensic	50
Hedex Seltzer	60
Cojene	95
Cough and Cold Remedies	
Coldrex	25
Cabdrivers decongestant	30
Do-Do (also listed for asthma)	30
Flurex	30
Tonics	
Effico	20.2
Koladex	21
Pro-plus	50
Yeast-vite	50
PRESCRIBED DRUGS	
Analgesics	
Hypon	10
Cafadol	30
Doloxene	30
Solpadeine	30
Syndol	30
Propain	30
Migraine Remedies	
Migril	50
Cafergot	100

SOURCES: *British National Formulary 1986.* OTC Index 1986.

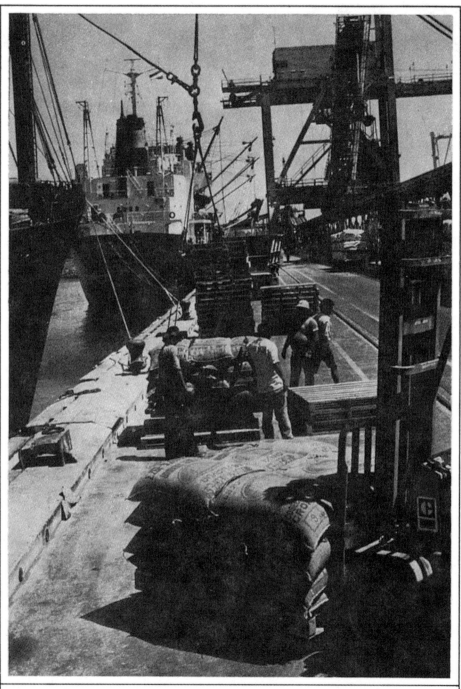

Sacks of coffee beans are loaded onto ships in San Salvador, El Salvador. In 1974 this Central American country was the world's fourth leading coffee exporter.

CHAPTER 5

TRADE IN COFFEE AND TEA

About 20% of the world's coffee harvest and 50% of the tea harvest are retained for local use. The remaining amounts of both crops are exported. International trade in coffee and tea is big business. The value of the coffee traded between countries, which is six times that of the tea trade, amounts to vast sums of money.

Coffee

Coffee is second to crude oil as an earner of foreign exchange for developing countries. Approximately 20% of all coffee is exported from Brazil, 15% from Colombia, and 7% from the Ivory Coast of the African continent. The chief importers are the United States (30%), West Germany (12%), and France (9%). Table 6 shows the average annual production and export of coffee from 1978 to 1980 by the dozen leading producing countries. Table 7 shows the average annual import during this same period by the dozen leading importing countries.

Trade in coffee is conducted mostly under the auspices of the International Coffee Organization, made up of 73 members—48 exporting countries and 25 importing countries. These countries are party to the International Coffee Agreement, which sets quarterly export quotas and regulates other aspects of the coffee trade. A new six-year agreement was signed in October 1983. The main objective of the current coffee agreement is to keep the price of a kilogram of green coffee beans constant.

Table 6

Production and Coffee Exports by Leading Producers*		
COUNTRY	ANNUAL PRODUCTION	ANNUAL EXPORTS
Brazil	1177	656
Colombia	702	633
Ivory Coast	242	230
Mexico	234	140
Indonesia	228	225
Ethiopia	189	80
El Salvador	159	151
Guatemala	150	134
Uganda	133	126
India	126	65
Philippines	114	15
Costa Rica	101	85
Other	1197	1121
World Total	4752	3661

*Averages for 1978–1980 in thousands of tonnes of green beans.

SOURCE: G.A. Spiller ed. *The Methylxanthine Beverages & Foods.* New York: Alan R. Liss, 1984.

Table 7

Annual Coffee Imports by Leading Importers*	
COUNTRY	IMPORTS
United States	1136
West Germany	450
France	317
Italy	214
Netherlands	155
Japan	150
Spain	118
Sweden	95
Belgium	91
Canada	85
United Kingdom	83
Finland	62
Other	752
World Total	3709

*Averages for 1978–1980 in thousands of tonnes of green beans.

SOURCE: G.A. Spiller ed. *The Methylxanthine Beverages & Foods.* New York: Alan R. Liss, 1984.

Overall, about 27% of the coffee trade is of the inferior and relatively caffeine-rich Robusta beans. The remainder consists of Arabica beans of a wide range of quality. Countries differ greatly in the kinds of beans they import. For example, 58% of the beans imported into France is Robusta, whereas less than 10% of the coffee imported into West Germany is Robusta.

Though world coffee consumption is changing little, production is increasing. This has created large surpluses of green coffee beans. These surpluses yield no income to pay for coffee-plantation workers or the materials they use. The temptation is to release more coffee on to the world's market, but this would depress the price of all coffee and possibly cause even greater problems for the producers. The International Coffee Agreement is designed precisely to strike a balance between these conflicting demands on the producers.

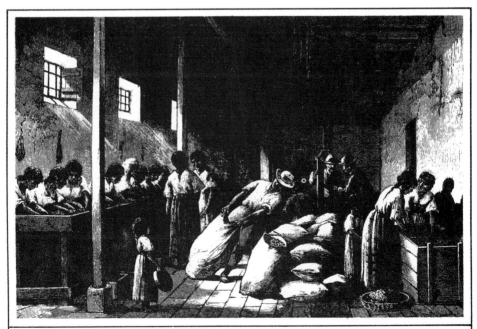

An 1882 woodcut depicts workers packing coffee in Costa Rica, one of 73 nations protected by the International Coffee Agreement, which ensures an economic balance between coffee producers and importers.

Tea

Tea is exported chiefly from India (averaging 26% of the annual total), Sri Lanka (22%) and China (13%). India and China are the major producers but retain much of their crop for local use (see Table 8). The major importing countries are Britain (23% of the total), the United States (9%) and Pakistan (8%) (see Table 9).

Trade in tea has not been internationally regulated since the 1930s. However, the supply and demand of the world market along with the governments of individual exporting countries have controlled trade. Demand, which usually runs ahead of supply, and the problems of storing tea for more than a few months make it difficult for exporters to control the market.

Opponents of regulation have stated that regulation is unnecessary because, when compared with other commodities, tea prices have been very stable. In 1984, however, tea prices were at record levels and rising at close to the rate of 100% a year. Discussions about the possibility of a new International Tea Agreement continue at the Food and Agriculture Organization.

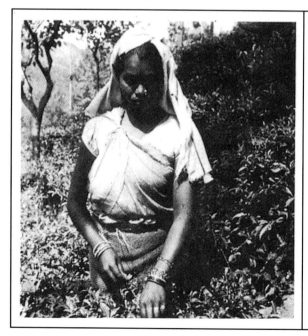

An Indian woman picks tea. India is the foremost tea-producing nation, accounting for over a quarter of the world's total production.

Table 8

Annual Production and Tea Exports by Leading Producers*		
COUNTRY	PRODUCTION	EXPORTS
India	565	200
China	329	121
Sri Lanka	205	187
Soviet Union	120	18
Japan	102	3
Kenya	94	91
Turkey	94	4
Indonesia	86	61
Bangladesh	37	27
Malawi	32	31
Argentina	29	30
Iran	25	1
Vietnam	21	8
Other	100	135
World Total	1837	917

*Averages for 1978–1980 in thousands of tonnes of leaf.

SOURCE: G.A. Spiller ed. *The Methylxanthine Beverages & Foods.* New York: Alan R. Liss, 1984.

Table 9

Annual Tea Imports by Leading Importers*	
COUNTRY	IMPORTS
United Kingdom	196
United States	77
Pakistan	60
Soviet Union	55
Egypt	30
Iraq	25
Australia	23
Poland	22
Canada	22
Netherlands	22
Iran	21
South Africa	17
Other	301
World Total	871

*Averages for 1978–1980 in thousands of tonnes of leaf.

SOURCE: G.A. Spiller ed. *The Methylxanthine Beverages & Foods.* New York: Alan R. Liss, 1984.

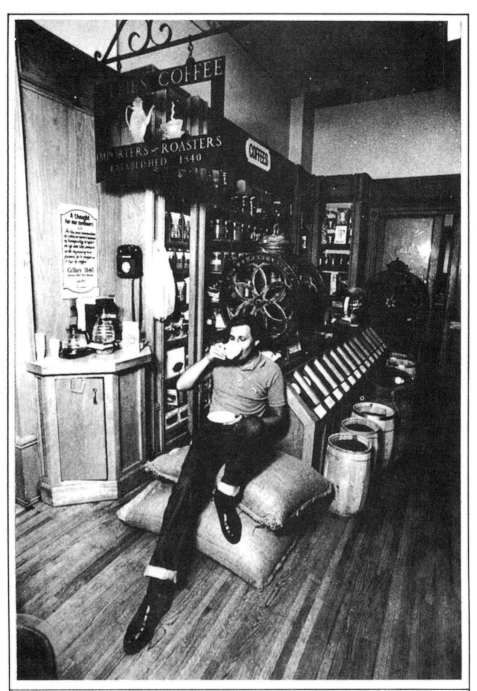

The owner of a coffee store in New York City takes a break amidst barrels, bins and antique grinders, Specialty stores such as this cater for the caffeine needs of sophisticated coffee drinkers.

CHAPTER 6

CAFFEINE CONSUMPTION

*T*he top ten countries with the highest per capita coffee consumption are in Western Europe (see Table 10). Canada and the United States, known as coffee-drinking countries, are in 11th and 12th place, far behind the four Scandinavian countries.

The decrease in consumption in 1977 reflects the high coffee prices that followed the devastating frosts in Brazil during the 1975–6 season. The wholesale price of a kilogram of green coffee beans during 1977 was more than ten times the average for 1971. However, the average wholesale price in 1980 had fallen again by almost two-thirds. In the United States the price of a pound of coffee doubled between 1976 and 1977. Only West Germany and Austria recorded higher consumption levels in 1977 than in 1970. Historically, these two countries have the highest retail coffee prices in the world and retailers were thus better able to absorb the increase in wholesale prices rather than pass them on to the consumer.

Though world coffee consumption generally declined in 1977, by 1980 it exceeded pre-1977 levels. However, not all countries showed an increase in consumption between 1970 and 1980. The Scandinavian countries and the United States exhibited an ongoing decline. This tendency is discussed later in this chapter.

Table 10

Average Annual Coffee Consumption*			
COUNTRY	1970	1977	1980
Finland	14.1	10.5	12.4
Sweden	13.2	8.6	11.9
Denmark	12.9	10.8	11.6
Norway	10.1	7.2	10.1
Belgium	6.6	5.7	8.9
Netherlands	7.0	5.5	8.7
West Germany	4.9	5.7	7.0
Austria	3.7	4.2	6.5
Switzerland	5.6	5.3	6.5
France	4.7	5.0	6.2
Canada	4.2	3.5	4.9
United States	6.2	4.3	4.7
Average consumption	7.8	6.4	8.3

*Per person in the 12 countries with the highest average consumption. Consumption is given in kilograms of green coffee beans or the equivalent in roast or instant coffee.

SOURCE: G.A. Spiller ed. *The Methylxanthine Beverages & Foods.* New York: Alan R. Liss, 1984.

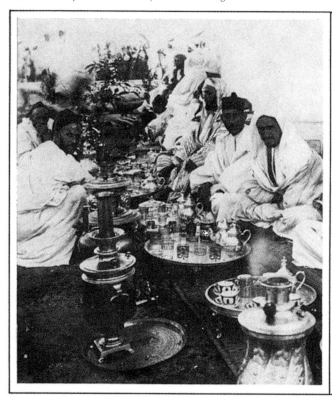

Casa Blanca, the famous Moorish café in Casablanca, Morocco. This is one of many establishments that serves coffee in the predominantly tea-consuming North African nations.

Table 11

Tea Leaf Consumption*		
COUNTRY	1974	1978
Qatar	4.2	5.9
Kuwait ,	3.2	5.2
Ireland	3.8	3.6
United Kingdom	3.5	3.1
Bahrain	2.6	2.2
New Zealand	2.5	2.4
Turkey	1.0	2.0
Hong Kong	1.5	1.8
Australia	2.0	1.7
Saudi Arabia	0.9	1.3
Sri Lanka	1.6	1.5
Tunisia	1.2	1.4
Average consumption	2.3	2.7

*Per person in the 12 countries with the highest average consumption.

SOURCE: G.A. Spiller ed. *The Methylxanthine Beverages & Foods.* New York: Alan R. Liss, 1984.

Tea Use in Major Consuming Countries

Of the twelve countries with the highest per capita tea consumption, six are or once were under British control (see Table 11). Five of the other six are Arabic speaking, and the remaining country, Turkey, has strong historical links with Arabian culture.

Tea manufacturers and wholesalers had hoped that the shortage of coffee in 1977 would increase the demand for tea, but this happened only to a slight extent. Because of this miscalculation, at the end of the year tea merchants were left with large stocks of tea. There is continuing growth in tea use in the world, but in general this is not because tea is being chosen over coffee. However, in some of the leading tea-using countries, notably the United Kingdom and Ireland, tea use is declining. On a per capita basis, no country is both a major consumer of coffee and a major consumer of tea.

Yerba Maté Consumption

The only other caffeine-containing substance consumed in comparable quantities to coffee and tea is yerba maté, which is used to make a drink known as maté or Paraguayan tea.

Yerba maté is consumed in quantity only in the five South American countries shown in Table 12.

The caffeine content of yerba maté is approximately one-third that of coffee beans and one-sixth that of tea leaves (see Table 1). Thus the caffeine intake per person from maté in any South American country is less than that from coffee or tea in any of the major coffee- or tea-drinking countries listed in the previous tables.

Table 13 summarizes the data related to world caffeine consumption. These estimates are based on trade data and take into account the caffeine content of the different items, the amounts held in stock, and the extent of wastage during production and storing. The estimate of "other" in the table includes caffeine from cocoa (about 1,350 tonnes of caffeine), maté (1,250 tonnes), chewed kola nuts and miscellaneous sources. World data does not include the caffeine consumed from caffeine-containing soft drinks. Because nearly all of this caffeine comes from coffee or tea, these data were included in the tea or coffee figures.

Caffeine consumption in the UK is among the highest in the world, six times the world average. All the countries listed on Table 13 have higher than average caffeine consumption levels.

Ranges in Caffeine-Beverage Use

Each day the British drink on average the equivalent of eight cups of tea and almost a serving each of coffee and chocolate. However, few people fit this average exactly, in caffeine use or very much else. In reality there is a wide range of consumption of each of the caffeine-containing beverages.

Given the fact that physical dependence on caffeine can occur when daily consumption of caffeine is in excess of about 350 mg (see Chapter 11), these data indicate that more than 50% of British adults may be dependent on this substance. And since regular use of more than about 650 mg of caffeine a day can pose a risk to health (see Chapter 12), approximately 20% of British adults may be in danger.

Table 12

				PER CAPITA CONSUMPTION
Yerba Maté Production, Trade, and Consumption (1977)*				
COUNTRY	PRODUCTION	EXPORTS	CONSUMPTION	(kg/year)
Paraguay	20	1	17	6.2
Uruguay	18	0	18	6.2
Argentina	143	4	139	5.4
Brazil	100	23	72	0.6
Chile	0	0	4	0.3
Totals	281	28	250	NA

*In thousands of tonnes.

SOURCE: G.A. Spiller ed. *The Methylxanthine Beverages & Foods.* New York: Alan R. Liss, 1984.

Table 13

	TOTAL CAFFEINE CONSUMPTION	PER CAPITA CONSUMPTION	
Caffeine Consumption in 1982			
COUNTRY AND CAFFEINE SOURCE	(tonnes)	(g/year)	(mg/day)
United States			
Coffee	10,300	46	125
Tea	2,850	13	35
Soft drinks	2,850	13	35
Cocoa	300	2	4
Other	1,000	5	12
Total	17,300	79	211
Canada			
Coffee	1,200	47	128
Tea	700	29	79
Soft drinks	150	6	16
Cocoa	30	1	3
Other	120	5	12
Total	2,200	88	238
Sweden			
Coffee	1,300	125	340
Tea	100	13	34
Other	150	20	51
Total	1,550	158	425
United Kingdom			
Coffee	1,700	32	84
Tea	6,500	118	320
Other	800	15	40
Total	9,000	165	444
World			
Coffee	64,500	14	38
Tea	51,500	11	30
Other	4,000	1	2
Total	120,000	26	70

SOURCE: G.A. Spiller ed. *The Methylxanthine Beverages & Foods.* New York: Alan R. Liss, 1984.

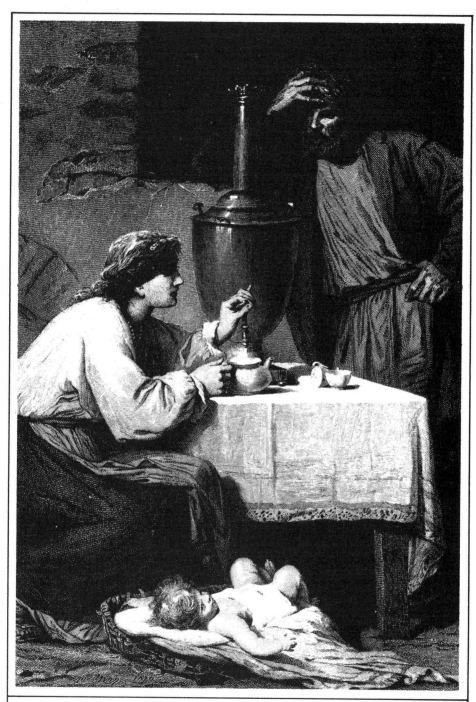

Tea-drinking rituals differ around the world. The woman in this Russian engraving, for example, is drawing the beverage from a samovar.

CHAPTER 7

CAFFEINE IN THE BODY

Drugs such as caffeine that affect behaviour and mood usually do so by acting on some of the 50 billion nerve cells in the brain. To reach the brain the molecules of a drug must first get into the bloodstream, which they do by a process known as *absorption.* This is accomplished in two basic ways. In *enteral administration,* caffeine's most common form of ingestion, the route includes the gastrointestinal tract — the mouth, throat, stomach, intestines and rectum.

Parenteral administration bypasses the gastrointestinal tract. Instead, the drug gets into the body via the lungs, skin, ear, or vagina, or by injection. Injections can be made directly into the artery or vein, into a muscle, into the spinal cord, or into some of the body's spaces, such as just under the skin or around the intestines. Though perhaps infrequently, caffeine has been administered through most of these routes.

Injection directly into the bloodstream is obviously the fastest route, but it is often the most dangerous. Some drugs, such as insulin, are not given enterally because they are destroyed by substances in the gastrointestinal tract. Other drugs, such as some of the barbiturates, cannot pass from the gastrointestinal tract into the blood vessels in the wall of the stomach and intestines. Therefore, these drugs are also not given enterally. And because the blood from the stomach and intestines goes to the liver before going to the brain, drugs such as cocaine and heroin, which are broken down very quickly by the liver, are also not effective if given enterally.

Because caffeine is not broken down by the acid in the stomach, it is readily absorbed by the blood vessels in the walls of the stomach and intestines. About one-sixth of a dose of caffeine is absorbed through the stomach walls, and most of the remainder is absorbed through the wall of the duodenum, the first section of the small intestine. In addition, caffeine is metabolized relatively slowly by the liver. These properties make it a suitable drug for enteral administration.

The speed with which caffeine gets from the mouth into the bloodstream depends on a number of factors. Absorption is slower, for example, when the stomach is full or after prolonged fasting. Usually a single dose of caffeine passes into the bloodstream within 30 minutes of administration.

Distribution and Doses

Blood containing caffeine flows from the gastrointestinal tract to the liver and then to the heart, from where it is circulated quickly throughout the body, including through the brain. The process whereby a drug spreads throughout the body is known as *distribution.* Caffeine is distributed to all of the body's water—approximately 42 litres, or 60% of total body weight, in an adult male. Of this 42 litres of water,

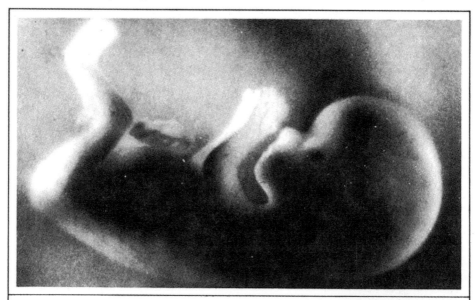

A normal 3-month human foetus. Children can be born with a caffeine dependency if their mothers continue to ingest the drug while pregnant.

only 6 litres is in the blood. Most of it—about 28 litres—is found in the cells of the body that make up the brain, muscles, and other tissues and the remainder is found between the cells. Because, unlike some drugs, caffeine is relatively insoluble in fat, it does not accumulate in body fat, a substance in which it could be stored for long periods.

The effect of a given amount of drug is directly related to the weight of the person or animal receiving the drug. This is because a heavier body will generally contain more water and therefore dilute a given drug dose more. The result is a lower drug concentration in the blood reaching the brain and the other organs where the drug has its effects. It is the drug's concentration in the blood that generally determines how strong an effect will be.

The relationship between dose, body weight and drug concentration in the blood is clarified further in Table 14. One must note that the caffeine-concentration levels would occur only if all of the caffeine dose were distributed evenly throughout the body's water *before* any of the drug had been metabolized by the liver. Usually concentration levels would be higher because uneven distribution causes more caffeine to be in the blood than in other body fluids.

Metabolism

Each time caffeine-containing blood passes through the liver, a small portion of the caffeine is metabolized. The caffeine removed from the blood is replaced by more of the drug returning from the body's other fluids. This process continues until eventually all of the caffeine has been metabolized by the liver.

Table 14

Body Weight and Dose and Blood Concentration of Caffeine		
BODY WEIGHT	154 lbs	184.8 lbs
Amount of caffeine administered (mg)	105.00	105.00
Effective caffeine dose (mg/kg)	1.50	1.25
Caffeine concentration in blood (mg/l)	2.50	2.10

The metabolism of caffeine is a complex process involving more than a dozen known metabolites, or products (see Chapter 3). Details of the process have become clear only during the last decade, brought on by the advent of powerful equipment for distinguishing closely related chemicals and by the development of sophisticated techniques for labelling parts of the caffeine molecule and tracing their fate in the body.

The main metabolite of caffeine metabolism is 1,5-dimethylxanthine, known as paraxanthine. During later passes through the liver the paraxanthine is metabolized, producing, among other chemicals, 1,methylxanthine, which is the main metabolite of caffeine excreted in urine.

The strength of caffeine's effect on the body depends largely on the concentration of the drug in the blood circulating through the brain. This concentration reaches a peak between 30 and 60 minutes after caffeine is taken by mouth, after most of the caffeine has been absorbed from the gastrointestinal tract, and before much of it is metabolized by the liver. (Caffeine's direct action on the brain is discussed in Chapter 9.)

Caffeine continues to have an effect as long as it remains in the blood. The critical factor is the metabolizing activity of substances in the liver known as enzymes. A lower rate of

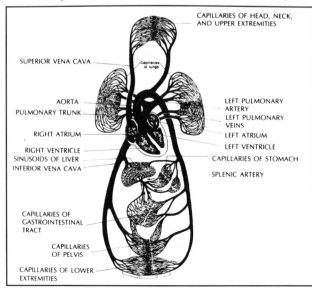

CAPILLARIES OF HEAD, NECK, AND UPPER EXTREMITIES

SUPERIOR VENA CAVA

Capillaries of lungs

AORTA
PULMONARY TRUNK

RIGHT ATRIUM

RIGHT VENTRICLE
SINUSOIDS OF LIVER
INFERIOR VENA CAVA

LEFT PULMONARY ARTERY
LEFT PULMONARY VEINS
LEFT ATRIUM
LEFT VENTRICLE
CAPILLARIES OF STOMACH
SPLENIC ARTERY

CAPILLARIES OF GASTROINTESTINAL TRACT

CAPILLARIES OF PELVIS

CAPILLARIES OF LOWER EXTREMITIES

Figure 4. *A schematic diagram of the human circulatory system shows how caffeine in the bloodstream goes from the gastrointestinal tract to the liver and then to the heart, from which it is circulated throughout the body and the brain in a process known as distribution.*

metabolism means the drug remains in the body and produces its effects longer. The half-life of caffeine—the amount of time it takes for the liver to remove half of the amount that has been ingested—varies considerably from individual to individual. The usual adult half-life ranges from 2½ to 10 hours, averaging about 4 hours. Most of the drug is removed from the body within 12 hours. Men and women tend to have similar average rates of caffeine metabolism, as do people of all ages. Because of the liver's role in caffeine metabolism, most kinds of liver disease, particularly liver disease related to alcohol abuse, increase caffeine half-life.

Use of other drugs can dramatically affect the rate of caffeine metabolism. On average, smokers, whose caffeine half-life is approximately 3 hours, metabolize caffeine 50% faster than nonsmokers. Thus, smokers experience the effect of a given cup of coffee for a shorter period of time than do nonsmokers. In addition, caffeine and nicotine have opposite effects on the neurotransmitter adenosine. Perhaps smokers tend to drink more coffee than nonsmokers in order to compensate for these effects.

Some drugs reduce the rate of caffeine metabolism. Alcohol has this effect, as does cimetidine, which is used to treat stomach ulcers. Use of oral contraceptives can more than triple the half-life of caffeine. Thus, women on the pill tend to react strongly to a second caffeine dose because residual caffeine from the earlier dose remains in the blood. As a result, these women tend to use less coffee and tea. Exposure to PCBs (polychlorinated biphenyls), considered to be major pollutants, also increases the rate of caffeine metabolism.

Some of the variability in rates of caffeine metabolism is inherited. Asians, for example, appear to metabolize caffeine differently and more slowly than Caucasians. Some of the variability, however, may be the result of experience with caffeine. Regular caffeine users may metabolize caffeine more quickly, though this has not yet been proved.

The rate of caffeine metabolism declines during pregnancy, particularly during the last few weeks. It returns to normal levels in the mother a few days after giving birth.

Women who are aware of the effects of caffeine, and this has been demonstrated in North America, tend to reduce their caffeine intake as pregnancy progresses. Most British women, however, whose caffeine intake is mainly from tea, do not reduce their caffeine consumption as much. Because caffeine metabolism is slowed, the amount of caffeine circulating in blood reaches high levels in many British pregnant women. Thus, the babies they are carrying receive high doses of caffeine.

Most of the enzymes that metabolize caffeine are not present in the livers of newborn babies. Caffeine in their blood has to be excreted through the urine, which is a slow process—the half-life of caffeine in newborn babies is approximately 85 hours. As the enzymes begin to be produced, the half-life decreases. At the age of 2 months the half-life is close to 27 hours, and by 4 months it is 14 hours. At 6 months the infant's caffeine half-life averages between 2 and 3 hours—below the adult level! It remains below the adult level until adolescence.

Paradoxically, the livers of newborn babies convert theophylline into caffeine more efficiently than do adult livers. As much as 75% of a dose of theophylline given to a newborn baby may be converted to caffeine, as compared to 6% for adults. Theophylline is used in the treatment of breathing problems in newborn babies, especially premature babies. The effectiveness of theophylline in treating breathing difficulties may depend on this conversion. In fact, some researchers have suggested that breathing problems in newborn babies may occur because the babies are no longer getting the caffeine they were used to receiving from their caffeine-consuming mothers. When a baby is breast-fed, it continues to ingest caffeine and thus avoids caffeine withdrawal. This is because the milk of a caffeine-using woman has a caffeine concentration of about 50% that of the mother's blood.

As well as being secreted into milk, caffeine is also secreted from blood into saliva and semen. Compared with the concentration in the user's blood, the concentration in his or her saliva is about 75%, and that in semen is about 100%, or approximately equal to the level in the blood.

Elimination

Except in newborn babies, there is very little *elimination* of unchanged caffeine. Only small amounts of unmetabolized caffeine are eliminated in faeces and in body fluids other than urine, and less than 3% of the ingested caffeine appears unchanged in urine. Most of the caffeine is excreted into the urine in the form of caffeine metabolites. This is done by the kidneys as the blood flows through them (see Figure 4) at a rate dependent on the amount of urine produced. Even though only a small amount of ingested caffeine appears in urine, the average concentration of caffeine found in urine is relatively high—about 40% higher than in blood—because the actual volume of urine is small compared with that of blood.

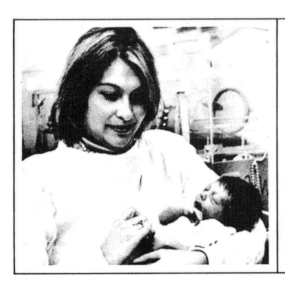

A mother holds her newborn baby. Caffeine received by infants before birth can remain in their system for as long as 85 hours after they are born.

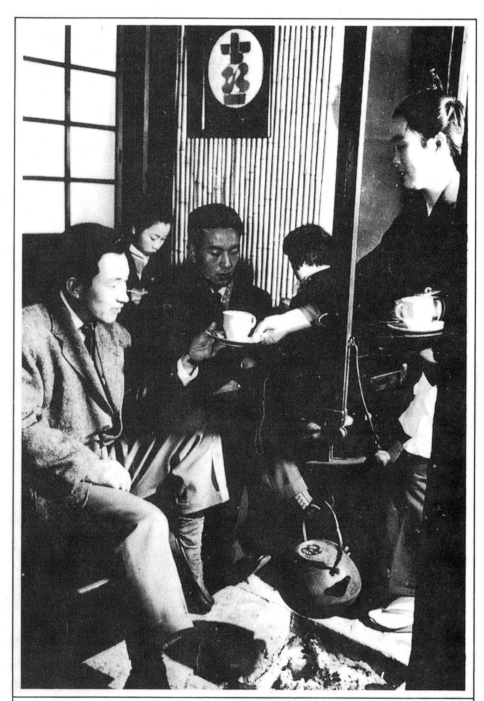

Customers are served in a Tokyo coffee shop as they warm their feet by the fire. In many parts of the world the partaking of coffee and tea is a ritualistic, often communal, event.

CHAPTER 8

VARIATION IN RESPONSE TO CAFFEINE

When people talk about the acute effects of caffeine, or those of any other drug, they usually focus on the desirable effects—at least when reference is being made to moderate doses. The acute effects of large amounts of a drug, however, are generally toxic and sometimes fatal. Mention of the chronic effects of a drug usually, but not always, refers to the undesirable effects.

Caffeine is used at least partly because of the short-term positive effects it is believed to cause in mood and behaviour. An understanding of what these effects are, and whether they even exist, may help one better understand why the use of caffeine-containing drinks has such an important place in human behaviour.

Knowledge of a drug's acute effects can lead to a more complete understanding of what causes the undesirable chronic effects. The chronic effects of a drug, including its contribution to certain diseases, is often the result of the body's repeated experience of the drug's acute effects. If one could show, for example, that every dose of caffeine has an effect on the heart, it could be determined whether caffeine use actually causes the heart disease with which it sometimes appears to be associated.

Why do some individuals appear to be more strongly affected by a given dose of the drug than others? Some people report that even a single cup of coffee in the evening disturbs their sleep. Others claim that before retiring they can drink several cups and experience few or no side effects. A number of factors explain this wide variation.

Tolerance

The most important factor contributing to individual variation in the acute effects of caffeine is *tolerance,* a condition that occurs with prolonged use of almost all drugs. Tolerance to a particular effect of a drug has occurred when the same dose of a drug no longer produces the effect it did initially. Thus, in order to achieve the original effect the dose must be increased.

Because repeated administration of a drug can reduce its acute effects, and even mask them entirely, studies of acute effects must use experimental subjects with no previous experience of caffeine—unless, of course, the study intends to focus on the acute effects of caffeine on tolerant subjects.

The observation that heavy users of caffeine require more of the drug to get them going in the morning is not necessarily evidence of tolerance to caffeine. These heavy users may have always been relatively insensitive to caffeine's effects. Tolerance is *acquired* insensitivity. Evidence for it can only come from observations of changes in the effects of caffeine with repeated use.

An example of tolerance to caffeine comes from a study of blood pressure in three groups of healthy adults. Reported in the medical literature in 1981, it remains one of the few studies of caffeine's effects in which factors affecting the development of tolerance were properly controlled. Group A (9 subjects) was given 250 mg of caffeine in a strong-tasting drink after they had abstained from caffeine for 24 days. Group B (9 subjects) abstained from caffeine for 24 days but received no caffeine in their strong-tasting drink. Group C (16 subjects) also received 250 mg of caffeine in the strong-

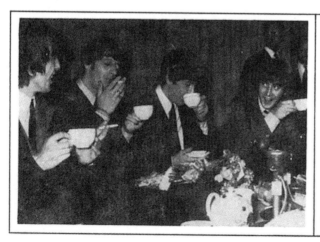

The Beatles at a press conference. Because of the effects of nicotine, smokers metabolize caffeine at a faster rate than do nonsmokers.

tasting drink, but they had continued to drink their regular three cups of coffee a day until 24 hours before the test.

All subjects received the strong-tasting drink three times a day for 6 days, and every day each subject's blood pressure was measured both before and two hours after the 9 a.m. administration of the drink.

The results indicate that in every subject, regardless of history or caffeine dosage, average blood pressure was higher after consuming the strong-tasting drink (see Figure 5). Clearly, something other than caffeine must have caused the increase. Perhaps each subject's blood pressure was normally higher at 11 a.m. than at 9 a.m. Whatever the reason, the changes in blood pressure in the subjects who received caffeine (those in Groups A and C) needed to be compared with this baseline increase.

That Bar A_1 is very much higher than Bar B_1 indicates that caffeine, ingested after 24 days of abstinence, initially produces a significant increase in blood pressure. However, on the fourth day of caffeine administration there was no difference between these two groups, indicating that complete tolerance to the effect of caffeine on blood pressure had developed in the subjects in Group A.

In analysing the results, Group C was split into two subgroups according to how much caffeine was found in the

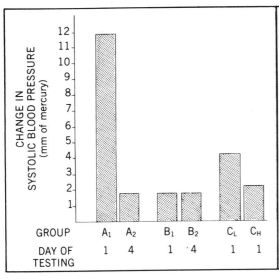

Figure 5. *A chart of a test in which members of groups A and C ingested 250 mg of caffeine. Results showed that persons in group A, who had abstained from the substance for 24 days, had significantly higher blood pressure the first day but by the fourth day had developed a tolerance so that their blood pressure was the same as members of group B, who ingested no caffeine. The pressure of those in group C (persons with a high tolerance for caffeine) was not affected significantly.*

subject's blood just prior to receiving the strong-tasting, caffeine-containing drink. Sub-group C_L had less than 1 mg of caffeine per litre of blood, indicating that these subjects usually drank weak coffee and/or that they metabolize caffeine quickly. As shown in Figure 5, the caffeine significantly increased the blood pressure of these subjects, though the increase was considerably less than that for the subjects in Group A, who had abstained from caffeine for 24 days rather than for 1 day.

Subjects in Sub-group C_H had more than 1 mg of caffeine per litre of blood when originally tested, indicating that they usually drank stronger coffee and/or metabolized caffeine slowly. Their blood pressure increased insignificantly after they consumed caffeine in the strong-tasting drink.

Three conclusions can be drawn from this study:

1.   A single 250-mg dose of caffeine can produce a significant increase in blood pressure in abstinent subjects.
2.   Within four days, repeated administration of caffeine produces significant tolerance to the effect of the drug on blood pressure.
3.   In some subjects, tolerance to caffeine's effect on blood pressure persists even after 24 hours of abstinence. In other subjects, one day's abstinence does reduce though

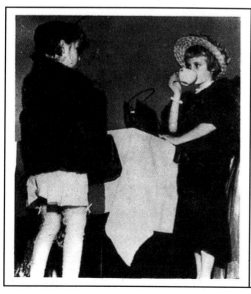

Dressed-up youngsters engage in a tea party. There is evidence that children who are exposed to caffeine before birth have a higher tolerance to the drug than those who have not been exposed.

does not entirely eliminate tolerance to these effects.

In this same study, the reasearchers also found evidence of tolerance to caffeine's acute effects on rate of breathing and on the amounts of certain chemicals in the blood and urine. Other studies have shown, with differing degrees of statistical significance, that tolerance can occur to caffeine's effects on urine and saliva production, on sleep, and, in animals, on general movement and on the activity of nerve cells in certain parts of the brain.

Because there have been few properly conducted studies of tolerance to caffeine, knowledge of caffeine's acute effects is uncertain. Many findings that caffeine has no effect on a particular function of the body may have occurred because the researchers were using subjects who were tolerant to that effect.

Other Sources of Variation

Even after differences in tolerance, rate of metabolism, rate of absorption and body weight are allowed for, there may still be causes of variation in response to caffeine. One additional source of variation may be found in the nervous system. For example, there may be inherited differences in the structure of the gaps between nerve cells that allow caffeine to compete more sucessfully for adenosine receptors in some individuals than in others. Such differences in the nervous system could explain the variations in response to caffeine with respect to personality that have been reported in the past (see Chapter 9).

Researchers who have compared children who use little caffeine (less than 50 mg/day) with children who use a lot (more than 500 mg/day) have suggested that the lower reactivity of the heavy users may be the result of exposure to maternal caffeine before birth.

The many possible sources of variation in individual responses to caffeine should always be considered when caffeine's effects are being discussed and investigated. The following chapters, which deal with caffeine's short-term effects, include much evidence that is contradictory, and this is probably because researchers have not paid careful enough attention to these sources of variation, particularly tolerance.

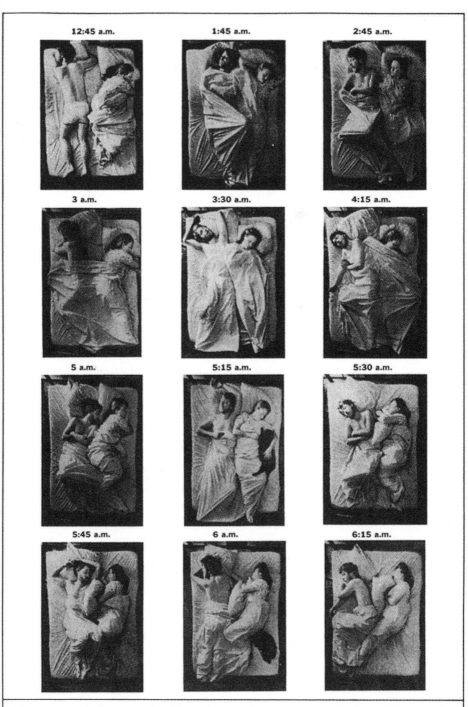

12:45 a.m.   **1:45 a.m.**   **2:45 a.m.**

3 a.m.   **3:30 a.m.**   **4:15 a.m.**

5 a.m.   **5:15 a.m.**   **5:30 a.m.**

5:45 a.m.   **6 a.m.**   **6:15 a.m.**

This series of photographs illustrates restless tossing and turning during the course of a night's sleep, a common complaint among caffeine users.

CHAPTER 9

CAFFEINE'S EFFECT ON THE BRAIN, BEHAVIOUR, MOOD AND SLEEP

*I*n textbooks of pharmacology—the branch of science that deals with the effects of drugs—caffeine is classified as a central nervous system stimulant. It is also known as an *analeptic drug,* or a substance that can restore strength, awaken and invigorate. This chapter is concerned with the various properties that give caffeine its reputation as a stimulant or analeptic drug.

There is little concrete knowledge about caffeine's effects on the brain, behaviour and mood at normal doses— i.e., between 40 and 300 mg. Thus, much of this chapter, which mostly focuses on the effects of doses within this range, consists of qualified statements and contradictions. While at times this may seem confusing, it reflects the state of caffeine research, a problem with which researchers too must contend.

Brain

Statements that caffeine stimulates the central nervous system—the brain and the spinal cord—are based on very little actual observation of the central nervous system itself. Mention of caffeine stimulation usually refers to the drug's stimulation of behaviour or mood. The assumption is that a certain degree of heightened brain activity is also involved.

Studies of changes in brain activity show that caffeine does have arousing effects. One way to measure this is to attach electrodes to a person's skull and record the patterns of electricity activity of his or her brain. It has been shown that the caffeine in a few cups of coffee causes the patterns to change from those typical of a resting, awake person to those typical of an alert and active person. Careful observation of the brains of animals have shown that caffeine enhances the activity of cells both at the surface of the cortex (that area of the brain associated with complex sensations and behaviour), and in the deeper structures of the brain (those areas associated with primitive behaviour and emotion).

As discussed in Chapter 3, the current theory is that caffeine interferes with the actions of the neurotransmitter adenosine. Though evidence in support of this theory is accumulating, because of the brain's complexity we are still a long way from explaining every feature of caffeine's actions on the central nervous system.

Behaviour

Apart from the effect on sleep, the clearest effect of regular doses of caffeine—equivalent to one or two average-strength and average-sized cups of coffee, or about 1½ mg caffeine

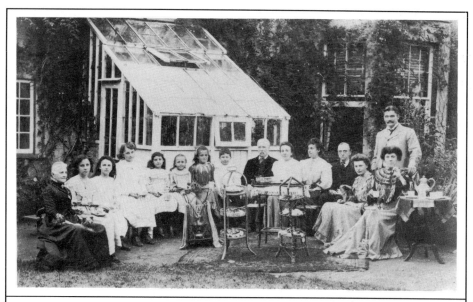

When the "taking" of afternoon tea was part of a social ritual often involving the whole family, as shown here in 1905, little thought would have been given to the effect of caffeine on the central nervous system.

per 1 kg of liquid—is an increase in general bodily movement. This has mostly been observed in animals, although when the right measurements are made this effect can also be seen in humans. However, even this most obvious effect on behaviour is sometimes not found. In fact, when researchers gave these relatively low doses of caffeine to experimental animals, occasionally *reductions* in general activity were observed. Almost all studies have found that animals receiving very high doses of caffeine (greater than about 50 mg/kg) show reduced general activity.

In humans, studies of caffeine's effects on activity have focused on work output and athletic performance. The usual finding is that the caffeine in two or three average cups of coffee prolongs the amount of time an individual can perform physically exhausting work. The quality of the physical work is *not* improved, except when the performance only depends on endurance, as in long-distance running, cross-country skiing and cycling. This effect on performance seems greater if the work load is constant rather than increasing, if the work is being done at a high altitude rather than at sea level and at normal rather than cold temperatures. Caffeine has also been shown to shorten the time needed to recover from exhausting work.

In Tibet, which lies between 12,000 feet (3657.60m) and 17,000 feet (5181.60m) above sea level, tea has been

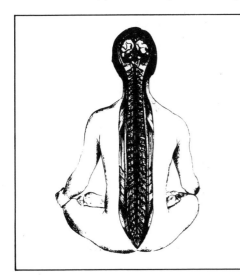

An illustration of the central nervous system. Caffeine is reputed to have stimulating effects on the brain and spinal cord, affecting behaviour, mood and possibly heightening brain activity.

used for centuries as an aid to endurance. According to William Emboden, the author of *Narcotic Plants,*

> *Weary horses and mules are given large vessels of tea to increase their capacity to work. Mules are said to be gamboling like colts as a result of their tea rations.... The distance between villages is accounted for in terms of the number of cups of tea necessary to sustain the person travelling that route. It has been ascertained that three cups of tea is equal to eight kilometres.*

How caffeine might enhance endurance is not understood. However, we know that the avoidance of exhaustion must involve a slowing down in the rate at which glycogen—a muscle's source of energy—is used up. Caffeine must either cause more efficient use of glycogen or facilitate greater use of energy sources external to muscles, such as body fat and

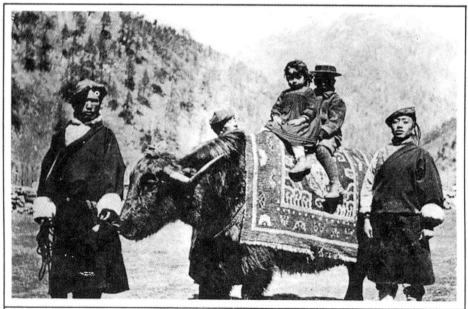

Travellers in Tibet use tea as an aid to endurance and as a measuring device: the distance between two places is gauged by the amount of tea needed for sustenance during the trek.

blood sugars. Preliminary research in this area suggests that caffeine acts both ways. Caffeine's effect on the body's use of energy is discussed further in the next chapter.

Some studies have found little or no significant enhancement of endurance by caffeine. Even a very small improvement, however, could make an important difference in athletic competition. An improvement by 0.6% in the time taken to run 10,000 metres might not be scientifically significant, but it would have reduced Alberto Cova's winning time at the 1984 Olympic Games in Los Angeles (actually 27.79 minutes) by enough for him to have broken the record of 27.64 minutes set by Lasse Virin at the 1972 games in Munich.

Athletes have, in fact, used caffeine to enhance their performance. Indeed, in 1962 caffeine was classified as a "doping agent" by the International Olympic Committee. It was removed from the list in 1972, but put back in time for the 1984 games. A 1982 study of 775 Belgian racing cyclists of many ages and levels of performance found that while their

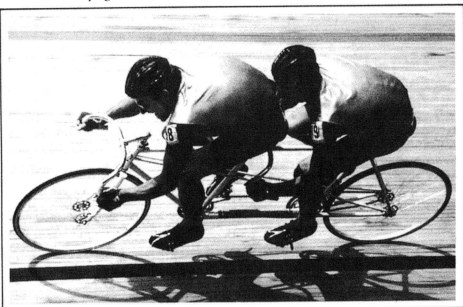

Two cyclists during a race. Because of caffeine's stimulating effects, the Olympic Committee declared the drug a "doping agent" in 1962 and again in 1984; an excessive dose of caffeine disqualified one athlete.

average regular caffeine use was lower than that of the general population, some professional cyclists were probably using excessive amounts of caffeine to help them in their races. The authors of this study suggested that caffeine levels in the urine in excess of 15 micrograms per millilitre should be considered evidence of caffeine doping. These levels could be achieved if an athlete drank three or four cups of strong coffee just before an event.

Where hand steadiness or fine motor coordination is required, rather than simple endurance, caffeine can cause a worsening of performance. For example, consumption of two or three cups of coffee has been found to reduce skill at needle threading and handwriting. Not all studies have found a negative effect of caffeine on this kind of behaviour, however. Some have actually shown an improvement. The question of whether caffeine has a consistent effect on skilled behaviour is still to be answered.

Caffeine disruption of fine motor coordination is ex-

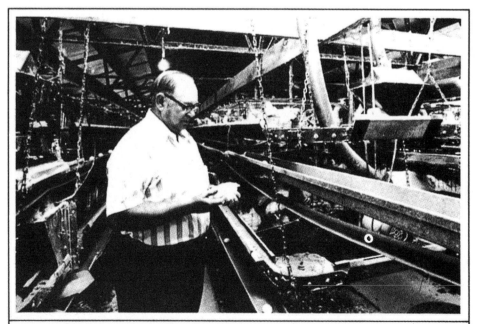

Some studies show that caffeine can improve performance of unchallenging, simple tasks such as egg inspection, which are highly repetitive and require long attention spans.

hibited as an increase in hand or arm tremors, sometimes called the "coffee shakes". Recent work, using equipment capable of detecting small, often invisible, movements, has confirmed the relationship between these effects and caffeine. At lower doses (150 mg) the drug may act only to enhance tremors already present and unrelated to caffeine use.

Perhaps the most interesting question about caffeine is whether it has an effect on intellectual activity. So far, unfortunately, research evidence based on performance ability appears to have many contradictions; much is based on categorization of personality types which is difficult to reliably and accurately measure. Because of this, the possible relationship between personality type and an individual's sensitivity to, metabolism of, and tolerance to caffeine makes research in this area very difficult and too complex for absolute conclusions.

Another question often asked about caffeine is whether it can counteract the adverse effects of drugs such as alcohol. In general, research in this area has also been inconclusive. With regards to caffeine and alcohol, both *synergistic effects* (when two drugs taken together produce effects greater than either drug alone) and *antagonistic effects* (when one drug counteracts the effects of another drug) have been observed.

In one recent study of reaction time, caffeine taken alone had no effect, alcohol increased reaction time (slowed the subject's response) and the caffeine/alcohol combination increased the reaction time even more. In another study, caffeine was found to counteract the negative effect of alcohol on the performance of mental arithmetic in male but not in female subjects. And a third study found that at low doses neither alcohol, nor caffeine, nor their combination had a measurable effects on skills involved in driving, though the subjects reported feeling impaired after taking alcohol and more alert ingesting caffeine.

Overall, the scientific evidence does not support the idea that a few cups of coffee will make a person fit to drive after three or four beers. In fact, the caffeine can make the driver more dangerous. By heightening alertness, it may make drivers *believe* they can do things that in fact they are not capable of doing. Instead of being sleepy, harmless drunks, they become wide-awake, dangerous drunks.

Similar confusion exists about the interactions between caffeine and other drugs, including marijuana and tranquillizers such as diazepam. Definite statements cannot be made because of the lack of clear evidence. However, it is always unwise to assume that caffeine will counteract the effects of any drug.

Mood .

Another claim made in advertisements, probably referring to caffeine's effects on mood, is that "coffee calms you down — and picks you up". Research into caffeine's effects on mood has mostly involved psychiatric patients (see Chapter 12), though there have been a few studies on the general population. The results of these tests have been contradictory. Use of moderate to large amounts of caffeine (300 mg

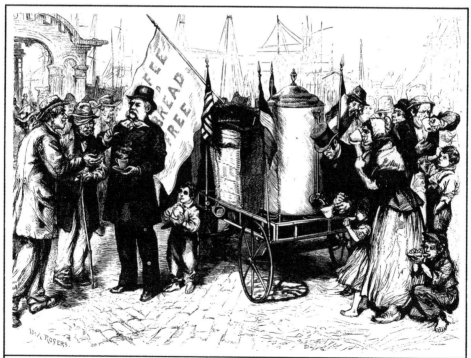

An old drawing shows temperance workers attempting to sober up the masses by serving them cups of hot coffee. Although caffeine is classified as a stimulant, it is not effective in counteracting the intoxicating effects of tranquillizers or alcohol.

caffeine or more) has generally been found to produce feelings of tension and anxiety, but not always. Enhanced alertness has often been reported, along with greater vigour and reduced fatigue, but again not always. Other mood effects also seem inconsistent, for example, depression and anger have been found to be both increased and reduced by caffeine.

These conflicting results may have occurred because the researchers did not take the regular caffeine use of their subjects into account. In one study in which proper account was taken, the researchers found that coffee drinkers experienced increased vigour and reduced fatigue, while noncoffee drinkers reported tension and anxiety. Another study involved children whose normal daily caffeine consumption was either less than 50 mg or more than 500 mg. The low consumers were more emotional and restless when they received about 200 mg caffeine. The high consumers were unaffected by the caffeine they received, but anxious and unaroused when they ingested a placebo. These children were probably dependent on caffeine (see Chapter 12).

Are the mood changes that follow caffeine use related to performance? Does caffeine make people work better because it makes them feel more alert, or do they feel more

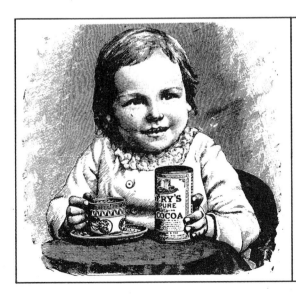

An engraving of a young child enjoying a cup of cocoa, a drink containing a low amount (about 2 mg per cup) of caffeine. Children whose daily caffeine intake is more than 500 mg are calmed and invigorated by the drug, but may also become dependent on it.

alert because they are working better? Again, the evidence is contradictory.

As with performance, caffeine's effects on mood can depend strongly on whether or not the subjects know they are ingesting caffeine. One study found that just being told that caffeine was being given enhanced both the feeling of increased vigour and the feeling of reduced fatigue.

Sleep

In contrast to what can be said about most of caffeine's effects on behaviour and mood, it is possible to say with some certainty that the caffeine in a strong cup of coffee consumed an hour before going to bed will have some effect on the sleep of most people. The noticeable effects are an increase in the time it takes to fall asleep and a reduction in total sleep time.

In a recent Japanese study, after ingesting 150 mg of caffeine, 8 subjects took an average of 126 minutes to get to sleep, compared with 29 minutes for those who had not consumed caffeine. The caffeine users slept for a total of 281 minutes, compared with 444 minutes for the noncaffeine users. Recordings of the electrical activity of the brain during sleep showed that the caffeine consistently altered the normal sleep patterns. These findings are similar to those of

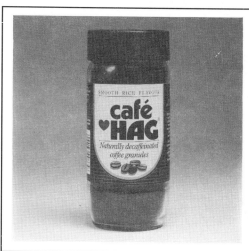

Ludwig Roselius, a German coffee merchant, first removed the caffeine from coffee and patented his process in 1906. The Kaffee Hag company was found in Bremen during the same year. Today, many people who like to drink coffee in the evening choose a decaffeinated brand to minimize the side effect of insomnia.

many other studies, although studies using non-Asian subjects usually produce less dramatic results.

Caffeine users are more readily aroused by sudden noises and exhibit an increase in body movements during sleep and a decrease in the reported quality of sleep. There is disagreement as to caffeine's effect on the phase of sleep known as REM, or rapid-eye-movement, sleep. Research has shown that it is during this phase, characterized by a specific type of electrical activity in the brain, that dreaming occurs. When caffeine is used, REM sleep tends to occur earlier, but researchers have not yet determined whether caffeine causes an increase, a reduction, or, in fact, any change in the quantity or quality of REM sleep and/or dreaming.

Although there are considerable differences in reactions to caffeine, people who consume a lot of caffeine usually sleep for shorter periods than people who use less. Therefore, heavy caffeine users may well suffer from some degree of chronic insomnia.

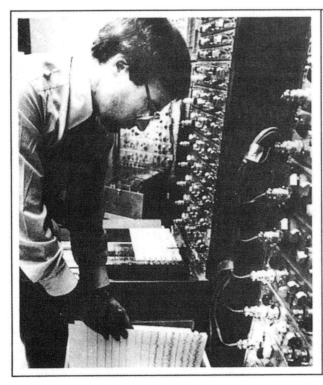

A researcher consults a chart depicting the influence of various drugs on the brain. Modern technology enables scientists to partially isolate a physical system in order to study the effects of a substance such as caffeine.

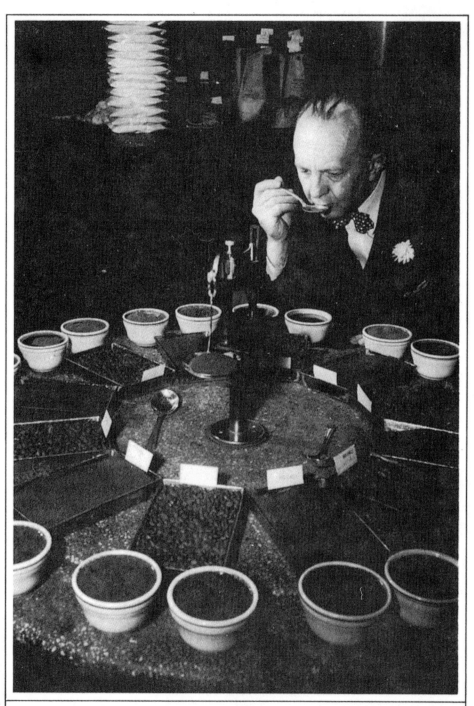

An inspector takes a sample from one of many cups of a coffee company's product. Taken in excess, caffeine can have toxic effects.

CHAPTER 10

⬛ EFFECTS OF CAFFEINE

⬛affeine reaches almost every part of the body and therefore has the potential to affect most of the body's functions. In fact, it does produce acute (short-term but often severe) effects on the cardiovascular system (the heart and blood vessels), on the digestive system, on breathing, on energy expenditure and on urination. This property has also made it possible for caffeine to contribute to the therapeutic treatment of illnesses and diseases. But in addition, this characteristic enables caffeine to exhibit its toxic effects throughout the body. At the extreme, caffeine use can even be fatal.

As mentioned in the previous two chapters, scientists studying the effects of caffeine on the human body have not been particularly careful to take into consideration the large differences between individual responses. Because of this there remains considerable uncertainty about caffeine's effects.

Cardiovascular Effects

Two important measures of cardiovascular function are the pressure of the blood as it flows through the arteries (blood pressure) and the heart rate. Blood pressure is of special concern because high blood pressure is an indication of strain on the heart and blood vessels and of possible obstruction somewhere in the circulatory system. Anything that causes or adds to high blood pressure could be dangerous.

A person's blood pressure at any given time depends on two things: the output of blood from the heart and the resistance of the circulatory system to the flow of blood. The output from the heart is determined in part by the rate at which the heart beats. When both the resistance to blood flow and the volume of blood pumped through the system at each heart beat remain constant, blood pressure and heart rate rise and fall together.

Caffeine significantly increases the blood pressure in subjects who have been without the drug for some days (see Chapter 8). Complete tolerance to this effect develops quickly. In the study discussed in Chapter 8, this occurred after four days.

When the 1981 study was repeated using slightly hypertensive subjects—subjects whose blood pressure was a little higher than normal—similar results were found. However, some research has found a reduction in blood pressure as a result of caffeine administration, while other research has found none at all. Moreover, although the weight of evidence points to a transient (i.e., short-lived) increase in blood pressure as the main result of caffeine use, there are recent reports that people who consume heavy amounts of coffee, even when they are not under the influence of caffeine, tend to have slightly higher blood pressure than people who use little or no coffee.

Increased heart rate usually accompanies the use of caffeine, although the change is generally small and not statistically significant. In some studies, including the one mentioned above on slightly hypertensive subjects, reduced heart rate was found after caffeine administration. Other researchers have reported that caffeine causes an initial decrease and then an increase in heart rate.

Similar confusion exists concerning caffeine's effects on the circulatory system's resistance to blood flow. Some researchers have found dilation (widening) of blood vessels, particularly those in the brain. But both constriction of and a lack of any effect on blood vessels have also been observed.

A recent concern has been the possible role of caffeine in the occurrence of arrhythmias—irregularities in the heart beat, sometimes known as palpitations. Forms of arrhythmias are thought to be involved in some cases of death from heart failure. A well-publicized experiment, reported in 1983, demonstrated that caffeine given orally or intravenously will reliably produce arrythmias in subjects who had previous arrhythmic symptoms.

Respiratory Effects

Caffeine has been shown to increase the rate of breathing by heightening the sensitivity of the part of the brain that responds to the level of carbon dioxide in the blood. Caffeine can improve the depth of breathing by strengthening the action of the diaphragm, which is the main muscle concerned with inhaling and exhaling (see Figure 6). One study has found that caffeine could be useful for people with lung disease who suffer from breathlessness.

Asthmatic patients have difficulty breathing because their bronchial passages become constricted. Theophylline (see Chapter 3) has long been used as a drug that dilates the bronchial passage and thus makes breathing easier for asthmatics. A recent comparison found that caffeine was also effective. However, the effective dose (10 mg/kg or the equivalent of about 9 average cups of coffee for an average-

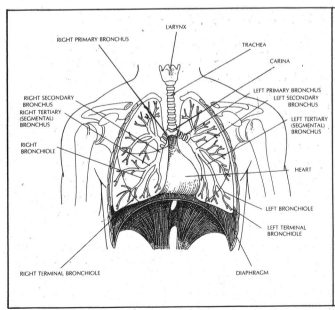

Figure 6. *A diagram of the respiratory system. Studies show that caffeine can improve breathing and relieve some respiratory ailments, but the amount needed to produce these results may also cause unwanted side effects.*

LARYNX

RIGHT PRIMARY BRONCHUS

TRACHEA

CARINA

LEFT PRIMARY BRONCHUS

RIGHT SECONDARY BRONCHUS

LEFT SECONDARY BRONCHUS

RIGHT TERTIARY (SEGMENTAL) BRONCHUS

LEFT TERTIARY (SEGMENTAL) BRONCHUS

RIGHT BRONCHIOLE

HEART

LEFT BRONCHIOLE

LEFT TERMINAL BRONCHIOLE

RIGHT TERMINAL BRONCHIOLE

DIAPHRAGM

size person) produced unwanted side effects in most patients, notably shakiness and tremors.

Energy Expenditure and Weight Loss

Caffeine's short-term effects on the body's use of energy might be of interest to people who wish to lose weight. When ingested with a meal, caffeine increases the rate at which the food is converted into usable energy. When caffeine is taken between meals, it causes fats to be transferred from deposits in the cells to the blood stream. Here, as *free fatty acids* they can be used as energy by most of the organs of the body.

Caffeine also raises the activity level of the body, which can mean that the energy derived from food is used up in exercise rather than being stored as fat. In addition, caffeine stimulates the temperature regulating centres of the body, which in turn produces an increase in body temperature. To sustain this change, energy that might have otherwise been deposited as fat is used. Thus, even when the body is at rest a greater amount of food is burned.

Caffeine is a common ingredient in nonprescription diet aids, sometimes also known as appetite suppressants. However, there is no evidence that caffeine does indeed reduce appetite for food.

Despite the apparent relationship between caffeine's effects and weight loss, and though regular caffeine administration to animals has been shown to contribute to their losing weight, still it is not clear whether, in the long term, caffeine use contributes to weight loss in humans. Even if caffeine proved to be a weight-loss aid, one must consider this drug's other effects before advocating its use for this purpose. Frequently a drug's negative side effects make its use highly undesirable and dangerous. In addition, for a weight-loss programme to be successful and lead to permanent weight loss, it must also include a change both in diet and life style.

Digestion and Excretion

Drinking coffee increases the secretion of acid into the stomach, but it may be that, in addition to caffeine, other coffee components produce this effect. Although caffeine stimulates acid secretion, it also reduces the peristaltic action of the stomach, the action that causes the emptying of the stomach's contents into the small intestine. Caffeine also slows down the passage of material through the small intestine, yet speeds its passage through the large intestine.

All of the above-mentioned effects can contribute to digestive upset, and even to ulcers of the stomach and small intestine. People who already suffer from digestive upset are usually advised to give up caffeine-containing drinks. In fact, there is evidence that these people are more strongly affected by caffeine than are healthy people. One study, for example, found that in normal subjects 250 mg of caffeine raised the rate at which the stomach secreted hydrochloric acid from 200 mg per hour to 2,000 mg per hour. This effect disappeared within 90 minutes. In patients with ulcers in the small intestine, the same amount of caffeine raised the acid secretion rate from 300 mg per hour to 4,700 mg per hour. After two hours, the rate was still above 3,000 mg per hour.

As well as these effects on the digestive system, coffee and tea also reduce the body's absorption of specific

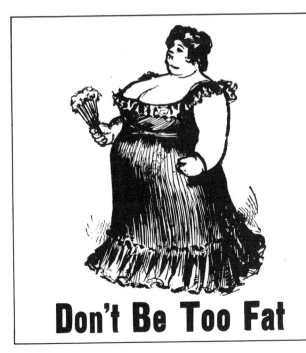

An early mail order advertisement promoting a drug-free weight-loss product. Many of today's over-the-counter diet aids contain substantial amounts of caffeine, which is not a proven appetite suppressant.

Don't Be Too Fat

nutrients, particularly iron, an essential mineral. The specific chemical or chemicals that cause the inhibition of iron uptake are not known, but caffeine and the tannins and other components of tea are the most likely agents. In addition, to this, caffeine's ability to increase urination—by 30% for up to three hours following ingestion—can cause significant increases in the excretion in urine of calcium, magnesium and sodium. Though some tolerance does develop to this effect, it could contribute to a deficiency in these minerals.

Caffeine as Medicine

Along with caffeine's beneficial effects on breathing, the drug is also successful in inducing breathing in newborn babies who experience breathing failure and continue to have spells of *apnea,* or cessation of breathing for more than 20 seconds. Caffeine drug also is effective in reducing the amount of apnea.

Caffeine is frequently included in both prescription and nonprescription headache preparations and other pain relievers (see Table 5). The amount is small—much less per tablet than in an average cup of coffee. Exactly why caffeine was

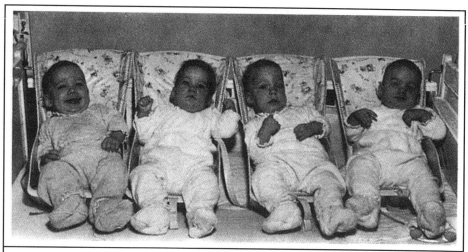

Research has suggested that caffeine, which is secreted into semen, increases the mobility of sperm and can therefore enhance fertility in some animals and humans.

first included in these products along with analgesic drugs (pain relievers) such as aspirin and paracetamol is not known, though it may have been added to counter possible depressant effects of these drugs. Caffeine may also have been included because it is especially effective as a remedy for headaches caused by caffeine withdrawal (see Chapter 12). But certainly few scientists and doctors originally assumed it was meant to increase the effectiveness of the painkillers. In fact, as recently as 1977 the US Food and Drug Administration issued a report that stated that there was no evidence that caffeine helped analgesics relieve pain.

Since that time, however, research has shown that the addition of caffeine does indeed increase an analgesic's effectiveness and reduces the time needed for the drug to take effect. When combined with caffeine, 30% less analgesic is needed. This characteristic of caffeine is true not only as regards headaches but with a wide variety of pains, including those from oral surgery and childbirth. How caffeine enhances analgesia is not known.

A small amount of research has suggested that caffeine may also enhance the much more potent analgesic effects of the opiate drugs, including morphine and heroin. However,

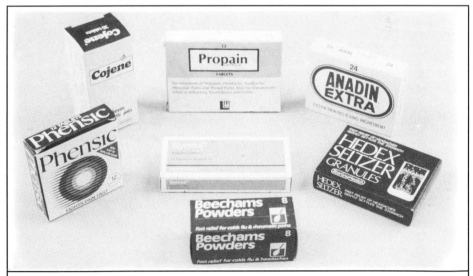

Despite the fact that caffeine is not a proven pain reliever, many prescriptions and nonprescription preparations contain a small amount of the drug.

to date, doctors have used caffeine only as an antidote for opiate overdoses. Injections of caffeine into an opiate user's muscles counteract the effects of opiate poisoning on the brain, and restore the user's breathing if it has failed.

Caffeine has also been used as an aid to fertility. A major cause of human infertility is sperm that are not mobile enough to reach and fertilize the egg. Studies of nonhuman mammals have shown that when caffeine is added to semen it can increase the mobility of their sperm and enhance fertilization. Studies of humans have produced similar findings regarding increased mobility, but until recently there had been controversy as to whether this led to enhanced fertility.

A recent study suggests that, in fact, fertility *is* enhanced by caffeine. According to the findings, women are twice as likely to become pregnant if prior to artificial insemination caffeine is added to the semen of their infertile mates. However, the concentration of caffeine used to achieve this effect is high—approximately 1,500 mg/litre, or more than three times the concentration of caffeine in the average cup of coffee approximately 436 mg/litre. The possible negative side effects of such high concentrations of caffeine used in this way are not yet known.

Caffeine as a Poison

Death from caffeine overdose has usually involved accidental administration by hospital personnel of caffeine by injection or by tablet, or suicide using caffeine-containing tablets. (One unusual case involved giving an enema of very strong coffee.) The lowest dose of caffeine known to have caused death in an adult is 3,200 mg, administered intravenously by a nurse who believed that the syringe contained another drug. Children have died from caffeine overdose after eating many wake-up, weight-control, or other caffeine-containing pills.

The acute fatal dose of caffeine taken by mouth is at least 5,000 mg—the equivalent of about 40 strong cups of coffee consumed in a very short period of time. Thus, death from a coffee "binge" is unlikely. Moreover, caffeine in high doses causes vomiting, which would add to the difficulty of consuming enough of the drink to cause death.

The actual cause of death from caffeine poisoning is not known, though in general the toxic (poisonous) effects of a drug are related to the drug's effects at lower doses. A wide variety of effects have been observed in patients who have received about 1,000 mg of caffeine, including the following:

1. abnormally fast or deep breathing (hyperventilation)
2. rapid heart beat (tachycardia)
3. involuntary, uncoordinated muscle contractions (convulsions)
4. rapid, uncoordinated twitching of the heart (ventricular fibrillation)
5. low levels of potassium in blood (hypokalemia)
6. high levels of blood sugar and ketone bodies in urine, as in diabetes (glycosuria and ketonuria)

The prolongation of any of these effects of large doses of caffeine can lead to death. Some doctors have noted that caffeine poisoning resembles the condition that can occur when diabetics do not take insulin or when their insulin fails to regulate the fat and glucose levels in their blood. Among diabetics this condition is the most common cause of early death.

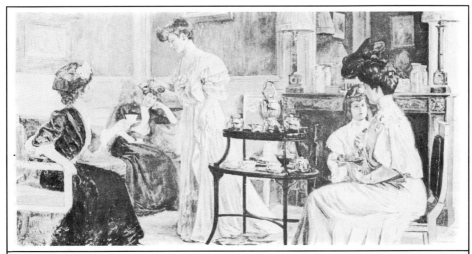

The afternoon ritual of a formal teatime was often simply an excuse for a fashion parade and idle gossip.

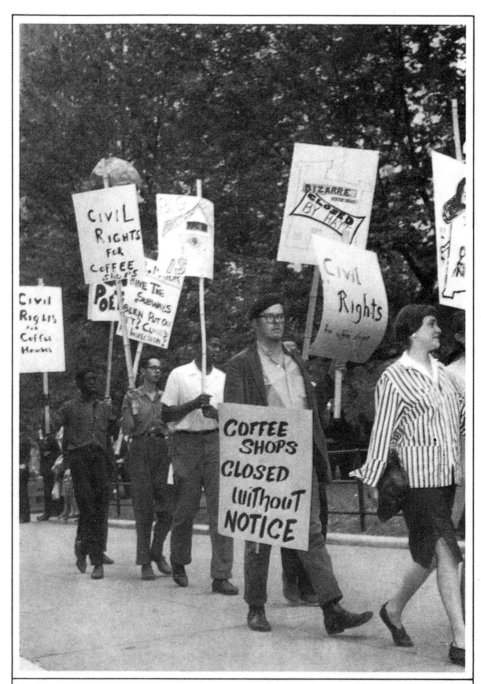

Members of the Beat Generation in New York City protest the closing of their favourite coffee houses. Drinking coffee was a communal pastime not only to the hippies of the 1960s but also to the turn-of-the-century bohemians, who drank it almost incessantly.

CHAPTER 11

DEPENDENCE ON CAFFEINE

A woman who regularly used more than 500 mg of caffeine per day was told to stop consuming this drug because it was causing irregularities in her heartbeat. She stopped many times, but on each occasion, after about 18 hours she developed a head pain, initially "behind the eyes" and "in the back of the head". The pain spread throughout her head, peaking three hours after onset as a "splitting headache", accompanied by a mild runny nose, moderate fatigue, and persistent yawning. During the headache she could smell coffee even when none was present. Aspirin alone did not help, but headache pills that included 65 mg of caffeine per tablet provided some relief.

One day, in desperation, she rapidly consumed two strong cups of coffee, or at least 240 mg of caffeine. Her headache and other withdrawal symptoms disappeared within 90 minutes, but her irregular heartbeat returned. She found that if she did not take caffeine in one form or another the headache would persist for at least 36 hours.

A man who regularly used about 1000 mg caffeine per day volunteered to take part in a study during which he was required to go without caffeine for 72 hours or more a number of times over a period of 6 months. He reported various symptoms of caffeine withdrawal at regular intervals during each of the 72-hour periods. Usually a headache developed first, beginning at about 6 hours after stopping, followed by fatigue, a runny nose, leg pains, sweating and then, at 16 hours, general muscle pains.

The symptoms increased in intensity throughout the 72-

hour period. The headache and leg pains were the most severe, followed closely by the muscle pains, with the other symptoms having moderate severity.

At 72 hours the man was given decaffeinated coffee. Sometimes with 115 mg of caffeine added. He did not know which he was being given. However, when he received caffeine the symptoms disappeared within 3 hours. Otherwise they continued.

These two case studies illustrate what is known as caffeine withdrawal, or the physical and psychological effects associated with the discontinuance of chronic caffeine use. The appearance of withdrawal symptoms is an indication that an individual has become physically dependent upon, or addicted to, a drug. Physical dependence, which may also include the tendency to increase drug dosage, is an adaptation of the body to the continued presence of a drug. Another type of dependence, psychological dependence, is a condi-

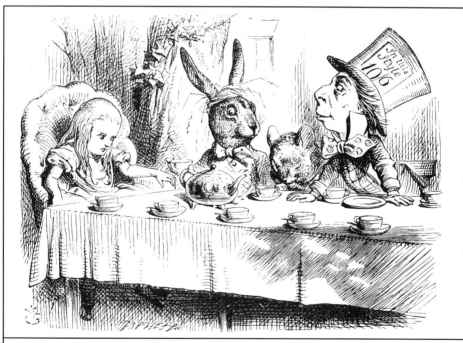

The Mad Hatter's Tea Party. An accepted scene from a traditional childrens' book, yet a few years prior to its publication William Corbett, author of The Vice of Tea Drinking, *wrote that tea was the ". . .debaucher of youth and a maker of misery for old age".*

tion in which the drug user craves a drug to maintain a sense of well-being and feels discomfort when deprived of it. Regular use of caffeine can produce both kinds of dependence.

Caffeine is capable of causing physical dependence in much the same way as other addictive drugs such as alcohol, heroin, nicotine and the barbiturates. But unlike the symptoms associated with the opiates, caffeine withdrawal symptoms, though uncomfortable, are not life-threatening.

One characteristic symptom of withdrawal not mentioned in the two case studies is anxiety. As previously mentioned (see Chapter 9), feelings of tension and anxiety can be produced by *giving* subjects 300 mg or more of caffeine. These same feelings may also be the result of *withholding* caffeine from a regular user. Because the effects of giving a drug and the effects of withdrawing from it are usually *opposite* in nature, further examination may show that, though the same term is used, the anxiety caused by caffeine stimulation may be rather different from the anxiety of caffeine withdrawal.

Though some heavy users appear to be able to cease taking caffeine without distress, there is very little evidence to support this. In fact, most heavy users are aware of the link between ceasing to use caffeine and severe withdrawal headaches and know that these headaches can be relieved by ingesting caffeine. Therefore, it is quite difficult for them to give up.

The lowest level of daily consumption at which physical dependence occurs is approximately 350 mg per day, or the equivalent of 4 medium-to-strong cups of coffee or eight cups of tea. It is likely that more than 50% or more of the British and other Europeans, aged 15 years and over use at least this amount daily (see Chapter 6). Physical dependence on caffeine is thus an endemic phenomenon.

Physical dependence is not inherently harmful. It can become harmful, however, when drug administration is discontinued and/or when drug doses become so great and excessively ingested that they can cause illness and disease. If, as in the case of caffeine (and heroin), dependence can be sustained at doses that may not cause harm, the only problem with dependence is maintaining the supply of the drug so as to avoid the unpleasantness of withdrawal. Generally speaking, caffeine use is a threat to the health of normal adults only when regular consumption is in excess of about 600 mg per day. Because caffeine dependence occurs after a daily dose of 350 mg, persons using between 350 mg and 600 mg of caffeine per day can be dependent on the drug without damaging their health.

Abstaining from caffeine, however, might very well pose a threat to the health of a dependent caffeine user. A person who uses a lot of caffeine and who skips his or her morning coffee could soon experience withdrawal symptoms. Such a person may be unusually irritable and thus accident-prone, socially disagreeable and inclined to self-medication, none of which is consistent with good health.

Many of the reasons heavy caffeine users give for liking coffee may have as much to do with avoidance of withdrawal symptoms as with coffee's virtues. A recent study found that coffee drinkers say the following things about their preferred beverage, in order of emphasis:

1. It gives you a feeling of well-being.
2. It calms your nerves and makes you relax.
3. It helps you think and helps orientate you.
4. It makes you less irritable.
5. It wakes you up and gets you going.
6. It reduces or avoids headache.
7. You would feel bad without it.
8. It stimulates you and gives you energy.

Caffeine is used to help newborn babies that experience apnea, or breathing difficulties (see Chapter 10). It is possible that some of these difficulties may be the result of caffeine withdrawal. Because their mothers used caffeine throughout pregnancy, at birth many babies will have already been exposed to caffeine. And if the baby is breast-fed, the supply of caffeine will continue after birth, In this way the baby's caffeine dependence is maintained. But if the baby is bottle fed, the caffeine supply ceases and withdrawal could occur, which could surely contribute to apnea.

The Theory of Caffeine Dependence

Craving for a caffeine-containing drink often appears specific to particular situations or particular times of the day. For example, a regular coffee drinker may drink a lot of coffee only in the morning and never in the afternoon or evening. Such a person may crave coffee in the mornings but feel no need for it at other times of the day.

This craving may be the result of psychological dependence on caffeine. Psychological dependence is a condition in which the user craves a drug to maintain a sense of well-being and feels discomfort when deprived of it. If this is the only type of dependence involved, one should be able to satisfy the craving by drinking decaffeinated coffee. If the craving induces a physical dependence, drinking decaffeinated coffee would not put off or alleviate the symptoms of caffeine withdrawal. Yet neither type of dependence explains why the lack of caffeine in the afternoon or evening does not lead to withdrawal symptoms.

Experiments with animals and humans have shown that tolerance to a drug can be specific to a particular environment. For example, a person might require less alcohol to become drunk in a strange place than he or she would in the place where alcohol is normally consumed. In this case the person develops a greater tolerance to alcohol when in the familiar environment. The mechanism that is involved is similar to what is called classical conditioning. For example, when a dog is presented with food, it automatically begins to salivate. If a bell is rung every time the dog is fed—thus associating the sound with the food—after a period of time the animal will salivate just at the ringing of the bell. This new relationship between the bell and salivation is the result of classical conditioning. Researchers think that tolerance, too, can be conditioned to be triggered by the events and objects in the environment at the time a drug is taken.

It is generally assumed that tolerance to and physical dependence on a drug go together. If this is true, since tolerance can be explained in part by conditioning, perhaps similar reasoning can be used to explain physical dependence.

Caffeine perks you up. The body, in response to caffeine—perhaps to protect itself from the effects of caffeine—becomes tired and lethargic. This state becomes conditioned to the environment, the events, and even the time of day associated with caffeine use. Thus, when the body is again in the situation in which caffeine is normally used, the conditioned responses of tiredness and lethargy are triggered. The caffeine user experiences these feelings until caffeine is taken. If no caffeine is available, the user suffers continued triggering of the unpleasant compensatory responses and experiences a range of withdrawal symptoms.

There is some evidence to support such a theory as it relates to tolerance, but little to show its relationship to drug dependence. However, the above-mentioned account should serve as an illustration of what researchers are thinking about when they attempt to explain drug, and specifically caffeine dependence.

Caffeine Hangover

As the 1960s had hippies, the late 19th and early 20th century had the bohemians. Members of this movement, which started in Paris and spread to other European and North American cities, adopted an easygoing, individualistic and sometimes eccentric life style which reflected their protest against or indifference to social conventions. *The Consumer Union Report on Licit and Illicit Drugs* said:

> *Like today's hippies, the turn-of-the-century bohemians were conspicuously drug-orientated. . . . In addition to alcohol, the bohemians used coffee. They drank vast quantities of this stimulant, were preoccupied with coffee, and suffered coffee as well as alcohol hangovers. Respectable citizens of that era were as horrified by the bohemian coffee cult as today's respectable citizens are horrified by marijuana smoking.*

Although caffeine hangovers are rarely mentioned in medical literature, there is reason to believe that the hangover that follows heavy caffeine use is as real as the hangover that follows heavy alcohol use. Just as the alcohol hangover can to some extent be relieved by more use of alcohol, the physical and emotional depression that sometimes follows a bout of excessive caffeine use can be relieved by use of more caffeine. Rapid intake of 3 or 4 cups of strong coffee (about 400 mg to 450 mg caffeine) provides a severe jolt to the nervous system that causes a high level of alertness and relief from fatigue. Then, some hours later, a headache, mental and physical depression, and feelings of exhaustion result.

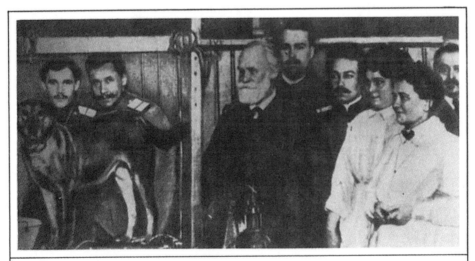

Tolerance to caffeine is caused by a process similar to "classical conditioning", discovered by Russian scientist Ivan Pavlov (centre).

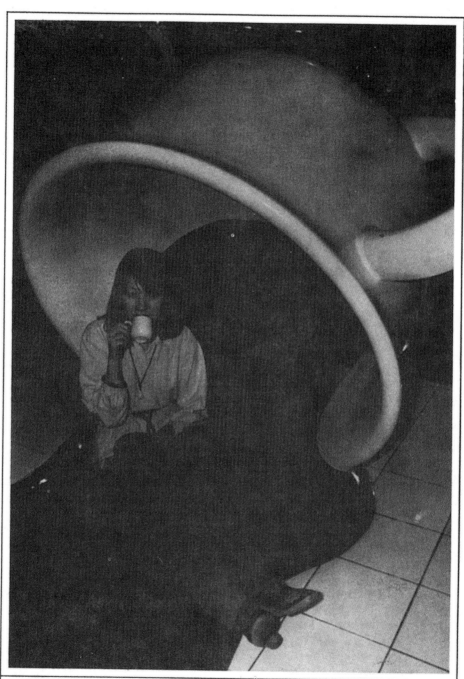

This oversized display in a Tokyo boutique emphasizes the prevalence of coffee in the daily routines of modern society. Although it is difficult to determine what the effects of chronic caffeine use are, sleeplessness and hangovers are known to occur frequently.

CHAPTER 12

EFFECTS OF CHRONIC USE OF CAFFEINE

*F*or well over a hundred years there has been medical and popular concern about the effects of the regular use of large amounts of caffeine-containing drinks on mental and physical health. In the late 18th century, William Corbett, author of *The Vice of Tea-Drinking,* wrote that tea drinking is "a destroyer of health, an enfeebler of the frame, a engenderer of effeminacy and laziness, a debaucher of youth and a maker of misery for old age".

In recent years interest has focused on caffeine's contribution to disease and death from heart conditions and cancer, and on caffeine's role in birth complications and defects. But in fact, there is currently no scientific evidence to suggest that regular use of moderate amounts of caffeine (up to 3 or 4 average cups of coffee per day, or up to about 300 mg of caffeine per day) is harmful to healthy adults. Of course, what constitutes a healthy dose varies according to body weight and many other factors. However, there are three instances that may possibly lead to complications: (1) when caffeine is used by a pregnant woman; (2) when caffeine is regularly consumed in the evening and causes chronic sleeplessness; and (3) when, within a short period of time, a large dose is taken and produces a caffeine hangover that makes the user ill each day.

A Note on Epidemiology

Epidemiology is the branch of medical science concerned with the causes and distribution of disease in populations. It deals with questions such as whether the chances of getting lung cancer increase with the number of cigarettes smoked, and whether the chances of getting typhoid are related to drinking contaminated water from a particular source. Epidemiologists look at a large group of people and attempt to determine how those with a disease differ from those free of the disease. In doing so they hope to be able to pinpoint the factors that could cause the disease.

Epidemiological studies do not by themselves provide scientific proof that a factor contributed to a disease. For example, just because heavy smokers exhibit a high incidence of lung cancer, one cannot immediately conclude that the heavy smoking *caused* the cancer. It might be because heavy smokers tend to live in cities rather than rural areas and it is the urban air pollution that causes lung cancer.

Obviously it is extremely important that epidemiologists consider all the variables and make allowances for them in experiments. In the smoking and lung cancer example, comparing heavy smokers living in cities only with light smokers living in cities would eliminate the variable of residence. But even when it seems that all factors have been

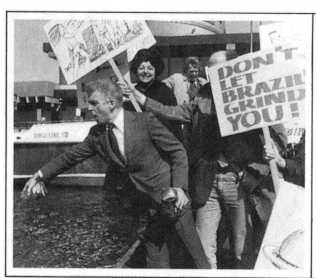

A group of demonstrators throw coffee into New York harbour to protest the sharp rise in Brazilian coffee export taxes, which rose by 500% in the late 1970s.

considered, there is always the possibility that some unknown variable is the real cause of the disease.

Scientific certainty comes from experiments in which researchers reliably demonstrate a cause-and-effect relationship. Experiments cannot be done in the case of human disease, because it would be regarded as wholly unethical for scientists to deliberately cause disease in human subjects. Most of our knowledge about the causes of disease, particularly diseases related to life style and drug use, must come from epidemiological work.

A major problem with this kind of research is that much of it relies heavily on reports by the very individuals whose habits are being studied. These reports can be vague or unreliable. Almost all epidemiological studies of caffeine use and disease have relied on information provided by subjects about their casual caffeine intake, generally given in terms of cups of coffee and tea per day. But, as mentioned in Chapter 4, there can be a six-fold range in the caffeine content of cups of coffee and an elevenfold range in the caffeine content of cups of tea.

The enormous variability in the meaning of responses to questions about caffeine use is enough to make it almost impossible to find precise relationships between caffeine use and the occurrence of disease. Researchers could develop more accurate indicators of caffeine use by examining blood-caffeine levels or by looking at coffee and tea purchasers, but this is usually not done. The general inaccuracy of measures of caffeine use makes it surprising that researchers are willing to give what seem to be unchallengable answers to questions about the extent to which caffeine use contributes to disease.

An important additional complication is the way in which high levels of caffeine use often accompany high levels of other activities, such as smoking, that can also cause disease. Unless researchers isolate caffeine use from other potentially hazardous behaviours, it will continue to be difficult to collect concrete information regarding caffeine's disease-causing effects.

Heart Disease

Heart disease is one of the main causes of death. The possibility that heavy caffeine use might contribute to heart disease has been a major cause of public concern.

Three important indicators for heart disease are high blood pressure, irregular heartbeat and high blood-cholesterol levels. Regarding blood pressure, caffeine has been found to increase blood pressure in subjects who have been without the drug for some days, but tolerance quickly develops to this effect (see Chapter 8 and 10). Thus, it is unlikely that caffeine would contribute to chronic high blood pressure.

Regarding irregular heartbeat, one experiment reported that caffeine produced arrythmias (heart beat irregularities) in subjects who had previous arrythmic symptoms (see Chapter 10). An earlier epidemiological study of 7,311 men

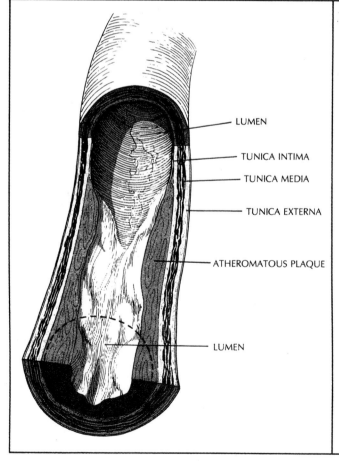

LUMEN

TUNICA INTIMA

TUNICA MEDIA

TUNICA EXTERNA

ATHEROMATOUS PLAQUE

LUMEN

A diagram of arteriosclerosis, a condition characterized by plaque deposits in arteries and that may be caused by, among other things, high cholesterol. Some studies have concluded that chronic caffeine use raises cholesterol levels in the blood.

aged 37 to 57 years found that heavy users of caffeine (more than 8 cups of coffee or tea per day) were more likely to exhibit ventricular premature beats, a type of heartbeat irregularity, than light users of caffeine (less than 2 cups a day). Because tobacco use, alcohol use and sleeping habits were among the controlled variables, they could be ruled out as having affected the results. Thus, irregularities in heartbeat associated with caffeine use may be one cause of heart disease.

Cholesterol is a fatty substance found in blood and in deposits on the walls of arteries. High blood-cholesterol levels are associated with hardening of the arteries, poor blood circulation and a tendency for clots to form that impair circulation to parts of the brain and may lead to a stroke.

In 1983 a Norwegian epidemiological study of nearly 15,000 people reported that cholesterol levels were significantly higher in subjects drinking more than 9 cups of coffee

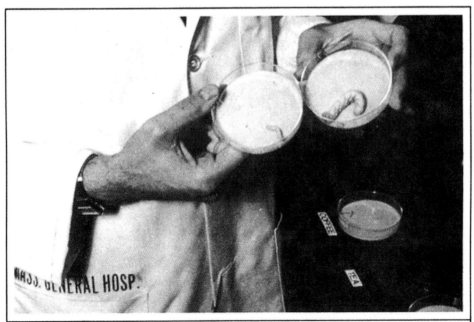

A scientist compares two dishes containing a normal hornworm (right), which was fed its usual diet, with a stunted hornworm which was fed a diet containing a significant amount of caffeine.

a day than in subjects drinking less than 1 cup a day. The researchers had controlled many other variables and thus were able to confidently conclude that coffee was a strong determinant of cholesterol levels in contemporary Norway. In addition, experiments with animals have found that when caffeine is added to their diet, their cholesterol levels are raised. However, epidemiological studies of North American populations have found no clear relation between caffeine use and cholesterol levels.

The Norwegian and North American studies of caffeine and cholesterol may have produced contradictory results because Norwegians tend to drink coffee containing more caffeine than North Americans. Once again, differing results may exist because what was considered a cup was not clearly enough defined.

Even though there is some evidence for the involvement of caffeine in the occurrence of both heartbeat irregularities and high cholesterol levels, the evidence relating caffeine and heart disease is generally minimal. Although epidemiological work in the early 1970s suggested a link between coffee use and heart disease, the link has not been confirmed by more recent investigations.

Another concern has been whether caffeine use can make worse a heart disease that already existed before a person started consuming caffeine. A recent study found that the caffeine in coffee actually delayed the onset of angina—a severe pain caused by a lack of oxygen in the heart muscle—and had no adverse effects on other measures of heart function.

The reasonable conclusion is that there is no clear and unchallengeable evidence supporting a link between caffeine and heart disease. However, because heavy caffeine use may be related to irregular heartbeats and high cholesterol levels—both indicators of heart disease—it is unwise to conclude that heavy caffeine use is *not* a cause of heart disease.

Cancer

The evidence connecting caffeine and cancer is also quite uncertain. A cancer occurs when cells of the body change in character, begin to divide uncontrollably and spread to various parts of the body. The change in the cells' character is known as *mutagenesis,* and substances that cause such a change are known as *mutagens.*

As mentioned in Chapter 3, caffeine can interfere with the way in which cells reproduce. Caffeine does this both by reacting directly with and by causing changes in the DNA molecules themselves, and also by interfering with the way DNA reproduces. In this respect caffeine is a mutagen.

Caffeine has been shown to be a mutagen in experimental studies at concentrations that are very much higher than those found in the body after normal caffeine use—typically about 200 times higher. Studies in which caffeine has been shown to be a mutagen have generally been conducted on the cells of bacteria, plants and insects, and on mammalian cells that have been induced to live and reproduce apart from the whole animal. It is important to note that a substance can change isolated cells without causing cancer in animals and humans.

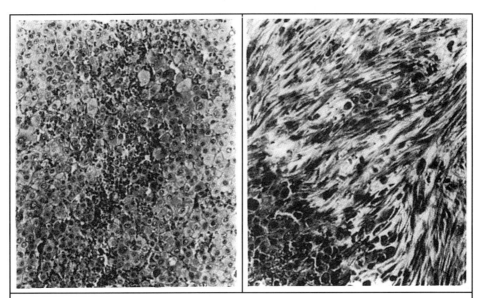

Microphotographs showing the growth of cancer in human tissues. Experiments concerning the correlation between caffeine and cancer have not proved conclusive. In some cases doses of the drug seemed to inhibit tumour production, at other times caffeine acted as a catalyst.

Lower concentrations of caffeine can enhance the mutagenic effects of other agents, but even these concentrations are at least 6 times the levels that would ever occur in a human body after caffeine-drink consumption.

Experimental studies on animals have generally *not* found evidence of tumour formation resulting from the long-term administration of high doses of caffeine. When caffeine has been given together with a known carcinogen, the results have been mixed. Large doses administered to animals under carefully controlled conditions have been found to enhance the ability of certain known carcinogens to cause tumours. Similar doses given under different conditions have been found to *inhibit* tumour production. Thus, in combination with known carcinogens, caffeine can be both a carcinogen and an anti-carcinogen.

In analysing animal studies, one must recognize the possibility that many of the results found in these studies may be irrelevant to studies of diseases in humans because of differences between the metabolism of caffeine in humans and in other species. In humans, the major intermediate metabolite of caffeine, paraxanthine, and the major excretion product, 1-methylxanthine, are both very similar in molecular structure to components of the DNA molecule. Accordingly, both of them may be more likely to interfere with cell reproduction than caffeine itself, although this has not been established. In rats the most important metabolite is a chemical known as 1,3,7-trimethyldihydrouric acid, also found in humans in small quantities. This chemical is *less* similar than the human caffeine metabolites to components of the genetic code. Thus, caffeine ingestion could be carcinogenic in humans and not in rats.

Epidemiological studies conducted in the 1960s and 1970s suggested links between caffeine-drink consumption and the development of cancer at the following sites: bladder, kidney, pancreas, colon, prostate gland, breast and ovary. Later and more carefully conducted studies have focused on cancers of the bladder and pancreas, and on cancerous and non-cancerous (benign) tumours of the breast.

Regarding bladder cancer, recent work tends to confirm a link between caffeine-drink consumption and deaths from cancer in men, but the evidence for a relationship in women is inconsistent. Positive associations, where found, have been weak but significant. It is reasonable to conclude that heavy coffee use (an average of more than 7 cups per day) can contribute to bladder cancer in men but not necessarily in women. However, overall rates of bladder cancer in women are considerably lower than those in men, making it more difficult to detect a positive relationship.

Recent work concerning pancreatic cancer has produced inconsistent results. Studies have both confirmed and contradicted an earlier finding that linked heavy coffee use and the development of cancer in the pancreas. A British study found an association between heavy use of tea and pancreatic cancer.

However, an epidemiological study can only identify relationships between variables. It cannot determine which of the linked variables is the one most likely to be the causative agent. Therefore, since it is known that damage to the pancreas can lead to increased fluid intake, it is not possible to say if the heavy caffeine use caused the pancreatic cancer or if the pancreatic cancer led to heavy caffeine-drink use.

A much publicized 1979 report suggested that benign breast tumours disappeared when caffeine was removed from the diet of women. Subsequent work provides data that do not support this finding, though a link cannot yet be ruled out. Although benign breast tumours can signal the later development of breast cancer, there has been little in the epidemiological studies to suggest a relationship between caffeine-drink use and breast cancer. Two recent experiments using rats found that the addition of caffeine to their diet enhanced the action of known carcinogens of breast cancer. However, one study found that caffeine tended to prevent the breast cancer in rats caused by the synthetic hormone diethylstilbestrol (DES) known as the morning-after-pill.

It should be noted that, in studies that found an association between caffeine-drink consumption and cancer, the caffeine itself may not be the cause of the cancer. In fact, both tea and coffee contain and are served with other substances that have been identified as mutagens. Therefore, further studies that eliminate the possible role of these other mutagens are needed before caffeine's true role can be known.

"Does caffeine use cause or contribute to cancer in humans? The answer, as yet, cannot be a clear 'yes' or 'no'".

Reproductive Problems

Caffeine can affect the unborn child in three distinct ways. Firstly, as an agent that can interfere with the reproduction of cells, caffeine could cause anomalies in sperm or ova, or in the way in which the fertilized ovum divides to form the developing embyro and then the foetus. Secondly, as a chemical that crosses the placenta, caffeine could directly affect the developing embryo or foetus in many of the ways in which it affects children or adults, or in ways that are especially harmful to an unborn child. And thirdly, caffeine could cause adverse effects in a mother that might have an impact on the development of the unborn child.

Studies in which animals are used as subjects suggest that all three of these things happen. Reviewing the evidence regarding caffeine's effects on reproduction, Beverly Mosher,

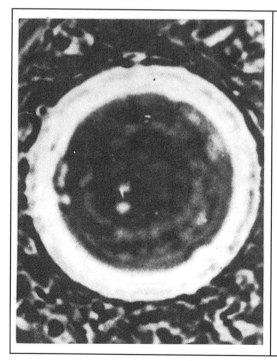

A microphotograph of a human ovum. For some individuals chronic use of caffeine can cause irregularities in the fertilized egg, resulting in possible damage to the foetus.

in her book *The health Effects of Caffeine,* concluded by saying that:

> *The studies reviewed ... clearly demonstrate that caffeine induces a variety of reproductive effects in several animal systems. Congenital anomalies and reproductive failures, such as reduced fertility, prematurity, low birthweight, and stillbirth have been demonstrated in mice, rats, rabbits, and chickens administered caffeine. Teratological effects [birth defects] include cleft palate, digital effects, jaw malformations, missing heart septa, and missing testes.*
>
> *However, animal tests may not accurately predict reproductive risk incurred by humans who consume caffeine. No firm guidelines exist for extrapolating from animal reproductive studies to humans. Hence, human reproductive risk cannot be reliably estimated from these animal data. Despite these limitations, attempts to define a no-adverse-effect level have been made. The level is considerably higher than all but the most extreme human consumption levels. However, certain individuals with a greater than average sensitivity to caffeine might also fall into a high-risk catergory.*

When it was written in 1981, the reviewer's conclusion fairly represented the then current knowledge. In addition to these findings, caffeine administered to animals during pregnancy had also been found to affect adversely the postnatal behaviour of the offspring. The main effect found in some studies was an increase in exploratory activity of offspring or in the general variability of their behaviour, neither of which is necessarily an adverse effect.

Because of the growing number of indications that caffeine could cause reproductive problems, the US Food and Drug Administration (FDA) began studying caffeine's effects in the 1970s. In 1978 an FDA committee recommended that caffeine be removed from the list of substances generally regarded as safe (the GRAS list). In 1980, prompted further by its own study of birth defects in rats, the FDA deleted caffeine from the GRAS list on an interim basis. Further tests were ordered, and pregnant women were advised "to avoid caffeine-containing food and drugs, or to use them sparingly". Canada's federal health department had issued a similar warning in 1979. In Britain, to date, no such warning has been given.

The first part of the FDA's own study involved the daily administration of large single doses of caffeine directly into the stomachs of pregnant rats. At doses above 25 mg/kg, birth defects—mainly toe or paw defects—were found in their offspring.

The second part of the FDA's study involved adding caffeine to the drinking water of pregnant rats. This experiment, reported in 1983, found no major defects even at the highest daily dose of 204.5 mg/kg although reduced birth weight and other problems were reported at doses of 86.6 mg/kg and higher. They reported no effects at or below 51 mg/kg.

Because caffeine administration in rats' drinking water is more like human caffeine-drink consumption than administration directly into the stomach by a tube, and because the former route was found to be less hazardous, in 1984 the FDA let it be known that its warning to pregnant women was being reassessed. Moderation may remain part of the FDA's advice, said a spokesman, because "caffeine is a drug no matter how you slice it. . . [Pregnant] women ought to limit their intake, but don't have to think they can't drink any caffeine or colas".

But how does one relate a daily dose of 50 mg/kg in rats' drinking water to a safe level for a pregnant woman? Some scientists have suggested that a 100:1 safety factor should be used in extrapolating the results of animal studies of birth defects. This would mean that the safe daily dose of caffeine for a pregnant woman would be 0.5 mg/kg—the caffeine in about half of an average cup of coffee. A second group of researchers has suggested that the correct conversion factor between rats and humans is 4:1, meaning that the safe daily dose for pregnant women would be the equivalent of about 7 strong cups of coffee. A third group of researchers believes that a 1:1 conversion is appropriate, meaning that the safety limit would be about 28 strong cups of coffee. If this were true pregnant women could essentially drink as much coffee as they pleased without adverse effect on their unborn children.

Studies of the relation between caffeine use and human birth defects and problems have generally not produced conclusive results. Part of the problem is that many pregnant women tend to reduce their caffeine use during pregnancy (see Chapter 7), making it difficult to find enough heavy caffeine users to make up a significant sample.

One recent study attempted to overcome this problem by interviewing 12,205 women about their coffee and tea consumption during the first three months of their pregnancies and relating this to the incidence of birth difficulties and defects. Only 595 of these women (4.9% of the total) reported drinking 4 or more cups of coffee per day. The babies of these heavy coffee users tended to be premature and lighter than average and were more likely to be born breech first rather than head first. However, this study failed

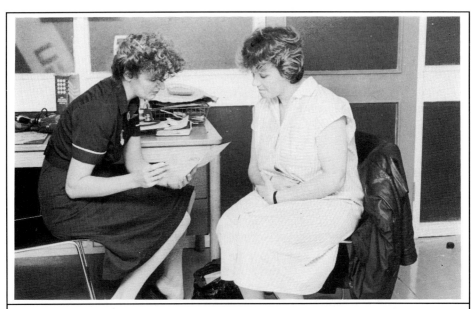

Medical staff should fully inform all pregnant women of the possible side effects from caffeine and other "harmless" drugs, if taken in excess.

to control for cigarette use, which was common among these heavy coffee drinkers.

Two other recent studies compared the caffeine use by women who had given birth to malformed infants with that of women who had had normal babies. In a US study that compared 2,030 such pairs, malformed infants were slightly more likely to have had mothers who had used some caffeine during pregnancy. However, the differences were not statistically significant and the estimated risk was not higher with high levels of caffeine use. A similar Finnish study involving 755 pairs showed no evidence of increased risk with caffeine use, even though average levels of consumption were very much higher than those in the United States.

One can only conclude that at the moment there is no direct evidence that high levels of caffeine ingested during pregnancy give rise to birth difficulties and defects. Evidence from animals studies, however, supports the conclusion that during pregnancy it is wise for women to be cautious about consuming caffeine in any form.

Behavioural Disorder: Caffeinism

Chronic excessive caffeine use has long been associated with abnormal behaviour. There was renewed interest in this possibility in the 1970s and early 1980s with the appearance of a number of reports that psychiatric patients with high levels of anxiety often drank a lot of coffee and could decrease their anxiety by reducing their caffeine intake.

In one study, for example, 22% of hospitalized psychiatric patients, whose scores on tests for anxiety and depression were significantly higher than normal, were found to be excessive users of caffeine (750 mg or more per day). In another study, 14 male psychiatric patients were, unknown to them or their nurses, given decaffeinated rather than regular coffee for 3 weeks. Tests showed a reduction in anxiety, irritability, suspiciousness and hostility. When regular coffee was introduced, previous levels of these psychological problems returned.

The syndrome, or group of symptoms, associated with excessive caffeine use is known as *caffeinism*. John Greden, psychiatrist, has written:

The most common anxiety manifestations of caffeineism are frequent urination (caffeine diuresis), jitteriness, tremulousness, agitation, irritability, muscle twitchings, lightheadedness, rapid breathing (tachypnea), rapid heart beat (tachycardia), cardiac palpitations (or skipped beats), upset stomach, loose stools and epigastric distress (heartburn and similar pains). Seldom do all occur together.... clinicians may find it impossible to differentiate the condition from anxiety neurosis or situational anxiety.

Many of these symptoms of caffeinism are consequences of the acute use of caffeine described in Chapters 10 and 11. The caffeinism syndrome appears to be a chronic problem because the patients are chronically anxious, i.e., they are anxious every day. But they may be anxious every day only because they use large amounts of caffeine every day.

Excessive caffeine use and stress have similar effects on the body. When they occur simultaneously their effects may be accumulative. Animal studies have shown that caffeine worsens both gastric ulceration and kidney disease when these conditions are caused by stress. Animals living in

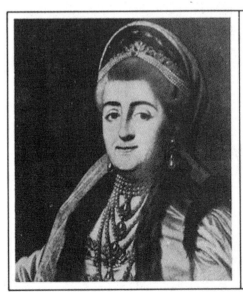

Portrait of Russia's Catherine the Great, whose personal imperial recipe for coffee consisted of one pound of ground coffee to four cups of water. The empress was known to be anxious and compulsive, symptoms often associated with heavy caffeine consumption.

crowded circumstances show increased aggression when given caffeine. However, caffeine has also been found to *reduce* aggressiveness in rats that have been in isolation.

In humans, the combination of caffeine and competitive stress has been reported to cause delirium. Caffeine and emotional stress have been reported as causing higher-than-usual levels of adrenaline in the body. Interestingly, increased caffeine-drink consumption can be a response to stress. One study found that female (but not male) college students used considerably more caffeine than normal during the week of ther final examinations. The combination could have caused serious interference with sleep and excessive stimulation, both of which could have interfered with good performance.

Caffeine has also been found to interfere with relaxation training, which is used to reduce a patient's reaction to stress. Caffeine-using subjects learned to relax just as easily as caffeine-free subjects, but, unlike the caffeine-free subjects, the caffeine users were unable to maintain a state of relaxation while viewing a stressful film.

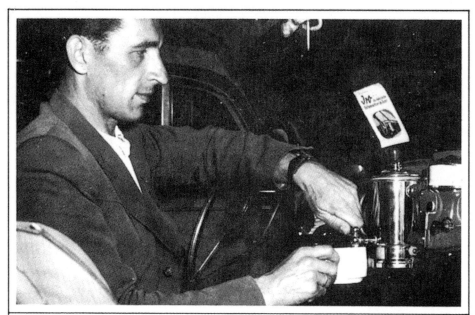

A small coffee maker, which plugs into the dashboard of a car, is indicative of the constant coffee intake in our fast-paced society.

One of the problems with treating caffeinism is that caffeine withdrawal itself can be stressful (see Chapter 11). A patient who is chronically anxious as a result of using caffeine may become more anxious when caffeine is withdrawn, and the anxiety may be made worse by a withdrawal headache.

Finally, the small amount of evidence specially related to children suggests that they respond to caffeine just as adults do. If children regularly use large doses of caffeine they can become chronically irritable, restless and anxious. These symptoms can also occur in asthmatic children who are being treated with large doses of theophylline.

Some children appear to be calmed rather than aroused by stimulant drugs. These children have been described as suffering from hyperactivity, hyperkinesis (excessive motor restlessness), attention deficit disorder, learning disabilities, or even brain dysfunction. One explanation of this paradox is that such children are hyperactive because their nervous systems are naturally under-aroused. In other words, they move around a lot, speak out, and are generally disruptive in class because they need to keep themselves from becoming lethargic or falling asleep. According to this theory, stimulant drugs provide this arousal of the nervous system, making the hyperactivity unnecessary. However, this theory is not based on actual measurements of the arousal levels of the nervous system of different adults and children.

Amphetamines, the stimulant drugs usually given to such children, are reported to help most hyperactive children. Some clinicians have used caffeine as an alternative. Experimental studies of caffeine's effectiveness have produced contradictory results. One study, for example, found that hyperactive children who used methylphenidate, a type of amphetamine, exhibited significantly improved behaviour, whereas caffeine (300 or 500 mg per day) produced no effect. Another study found that a lower dose of caffeine (about 150 mg) together with a low dose of methylphenidate (10 mg) was more effective than the low dose of methylphenidate alone, while a higher dose of caffeine (about 300 mg) with the methylphenidate dose was not effective in improving behaviour.

Thus, one can see that though caffeine can calm some children, it makes most children more restless, irritable and anxious. Clearly, more research is necessary before caffeine can be used to provide consistent and predictable responses in children.

Hazardous Levels of Chronic Caffeine Use

According to studies mentioned in this chapter, regular use of more than about 650 mg of caffeine (8 or more cups of coffee per day) may be associated with higher incidences of ventricular premature heartbeats (irregular heartbeats), high levels of cholesterol, bladder cancer (in men) and behavioural disorders. And while some researchers consider this dose as the maximum which can be used safely by a pregnant woman, many others have argued for a lower level and a few have argued for a higher level.

Given the most current evidence, it is reasonable to conclude that, in general, healthy adults may consume up to 600 mg of caffeine per day without doing themselves harm. As mentioned earlier, caffeine use during pregnancy, use that

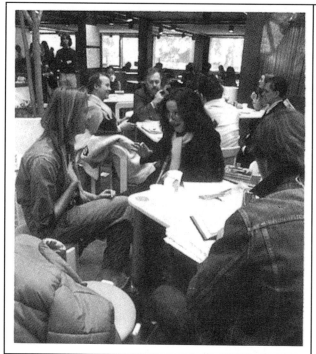

College women enjoy a cup of coffee between classes. According to one study, female college students used much higher amounts of caffeine during the stressful week of examinations than did their male counterparts.

leads to chronic sleeplessness, and use of high doses that lead to hangover may be exceptions. Also, it follows that since physical dependence on caffeine can occur at doses of approximately 400 mg per day, a person may be dependent on caffeine without necessarily being at risk of being affected by the various diseases that have been associated with caffeine use.

Approximately 20% of British people aged 15 years and over, or at least 10 million people, use 650 mg or more caffeine per day and thus are putting themselves at risk. Another 30 million or so have some kind of dependence on caffeine, a condition which may or may not be hazardous.

The risk from excessive caffeine use should not be exaggerated. Although it is possible to say with some confidence that excessive caffeine use is harmful, the harm is probably slight compared with that resulting from excessive use of alcohol or almost any use of tobacco.

Conclusion

Because caffeine is a relatively weak drug, but one that affects many parts of the body, sorting out the various consequences of using it have presented researchers with special difficulties. When humans are being studied, these difficulties are compounded by the pervasiveness of caffeine in our society. Because almost everyone uses caffeine and has experienced its effects, there are few unbiased or naive subjects.

Caffeine is used for its beneficial short-term effects—usually to maintain or increase alertness and to enhance physical endurance. Every other British adult may be dependent on caffeine and use it at least in part to ward off withdrawal symptoms. And about 1 in 5 adults may regularly use enough caffeine to cause physical harm, notably heart disease, bladder cancer in males and behavioural disorders. Of special concern is the possibility that caffeine used during pregnancy may cause or contribute to birth defects and difficulties. This possibility led the US Food and Drug Administration to delete caffeine in 1980 from the list of drugs generally regarded as safe. Caffeine is a drug, and though present data regarding its safety may be inconclusive, it is wise to use it cautiously and in moderation.

Some Useful Addresses

In the United Kingdom:

Advisory Council on the Misuse of Drugs
c/o Home Office, Queen Anne's Gate, London SW1H 9AT.

British Association for Counselling
87a Sheep Street, Rugby, Warwicks CV21 3BX.

Department of Education and Science
Elizabeth House, York Road, London SE1 7PH.

Health Education Council
78 New Oxford Street, London WC1A 1AH.

Home Office Drugs Branch
Queen Anne's Gate, London SW1H 9AT.

Institute for the Study of Drug Dependence
1–4 Hatton Place, Hatton Garden, London EC1N 8ND.

Medical Research Council
20 Park Crescent, London W1N 4AL.

Narcotics Anonymous
PO Box 246, c/o 47 Milman Street, London SW10.

National Association of Young People's
  Counselling and Advisory Services
17–23 Albion Street, Leicester LE1 6GD.

Northern Ireland Department of Health and Social Services
Upper Newtownwards Road, Belfast BT4 3SF.

Release
1 Elgin Avenue, London W9.

Scottish Health Education Unit
21 Lansdowne Crescent, Edinburgh EH12 5EH.

Scottish Home and Health Department
St Andrews House, Edinburgh EH1 3DE.

Standing Conference on Drug Abuse
1–4 Hatton Place, Hatton Garden, London EC1N 8ND.

Teachers Advisory Council on Alcohol and Drug Education
2 Mount Street, Manchester M2 5NG.

In Australia:

Department of Health
PO Box 100, Wooden ACT, Australia 2606.

In New Zealand:

Drug Advisory Committee
Department of Health, PO Box 5013, Wellington.

Drug Dependence
11–23 Sturdee Street, Wellington.

Drug Dependency Clinic
393 Great North Road, Grey Lynn, Auckland.

Medical Services and Drug Control
Department of Health, PO Box 5013, Wellington.

National Drug Intelligence Bureau
Police Department, Private Bag, Wellington.

In South Africa:

South African National Council on Alcoholism and Drug
    Dependence (SANCA)
National Office, PO Box 10134, Johannesburg 2000.

A number of organizations in South Africa provide information and services in the field of drug dependence. SANCA will
supply information on these, as will the government's
Department of Health and Welfare.

Further Reading

Brecher, Edward M., and the Editors of *Consumer Reports*. *Licit and Illicit Drugs, The Consumer Union Report on Narcotics, Stimulants, Depressants, Inhalants, Hallucinogens, and Marijuana—including Caffeine, Nicotine, & Alcohol*. Mount Vernon, New York: Consumers Union, 1972.

Dews, Peter B., ed. *Caffeine*. Berlin, Germany: Springer-Verlag, 1984.

Ford, Cathy and Sturmanis, Dona. *The Coffee Lover's Handbook*. Vancouver, Canada: Intermedia Press, 1979.

Goulart, Frances Sheridan. *The Caffeine Book: A User's and Abuser's Guide*. New York: Dodd, Mead & Company, 1984.

MacMahon, Brian and Sugimura, Takashi, eds. *Coffee and Health*. Cold Spring Harbour, New York: Laboratory of Cold Spring Harbour, 1984.

Mosher, Beverly A. *The Health Effects of Caffeine*. New York: The American Council on Science and Health, 1981.

Quinn, James P., ed. *Tea and Coffee Buyer's Guide*. Whiteside, New York: Tea & Coffee Trade Journal, 1984.

Spiller, Gene A., ed *The Methylxanthine Beverages and Foods: Chemistry, Consumption, and Health Effects*. New York: Alan R. Liss. 1984.

Weinreich, Moira. *The Tea Lover's Handbook*. Vancouver, Canada: Intermedia Press, 1980.

Glossary

adenine   one of the four purines that make up the genetic code in DNA

adrenaline   epinephrine; a hormone produced by the adrenal gland that increases blood pressure and is used in the treatment of asthma

amphetamine   a drug that stimulates the nervous system; generally used as a mood elevator, energizer, antidepressant, and appetite depressant

analeptic drug   a drug that acts as a stimulant on the central nervous system

analgesic   a drug that produces an insensitivity to pain without loss of consciousness

angina   a violent surge of pain usually caused by disease of the coronary arteries and degeneration of the heart muscle

anorexia nervosa   a pathological loss of appetite due to psychological problems and characterized by excessive weight loss and nutritional deficiences

antagonistic effect   the occurrence of one drug's effects counteracting another drug's effects

antipyretic   a drug that reduces fever

apnea   cessation of breathing for more than 20 seconds

arrythmias   palpitations, or irregularities in heartbeat

aspirin   acetylsalicylic acid; an analgesic, antipyretic, and anti-inflammatory agent originally derived from plants

barbiturate   a drug that causes depression of the central nervous system, generally used to reduce anxiety or to induce euphoria

cacao pods   the pods from the tree *Theobroma cacao*   which contain seeds used to produce cocoa, chocolate, and cocoa butter

caffeine   trimethylxanthine; a central nervous system stimulant found in coffee, tea, kola nuts, cacoa pods, mate, yaupon, guarana, and yoco

caffeinism   the syndrome associated with excessive caffeine ingestion; characterized by frequent urination, jitteriness, agitation, irritability, muscle twitching, lightheadedness, rapid breathing, rapid heartbeat, heart palpitations, upset stomach, diarrhoea, and/or heartburn

cardiovascular system   the system of the body that includes the heart and blood vessels

cholesterol a fatty substance found in blood and in deposits on the walls of arteries; high levels are associated with hardening of the arteries, poor blood circulation, and a tendency to form clots that can lead to a stroke

convulsion an unnatural, violent, and involuntary contraction or series of contractions of the muscles

cytosine one of the four basic letters of the genetic code in DNA

diazepam an antianxiety tranquillizer

dimethylxanthine a xanthine molecule that has two methyl groups; e.g. theobromine and theophylline

DNA deoxyribonucleic acid; a highly coiled molecule, or helix, composed of two long strands linked by adenine, guanine, cytosine, and thymine, which make up the genetic code

enteral administration a form of drug ingestion whose route of administration includes the gastrointestinal tract—the mouth, throat, stomach, intestines, and rectum

enzyme a protein that acts as a catalyst to chemical reactions

epidemiology a science that deals with the incidence, distribution, and control of disease in a population

fermentation a chemical process by which yeast consumes sugars, such as those in fruits, and produces effervescence and alcohol

free fatty acids fat cells that move freely within the blood and can be used for energy by most bodily organs

gastrointestinal tract the mouth, throat, stomach, intestines, and rectum

gene sequences of purine triplets within the DNA molecule that code all hereditary traits

glycogen a complex sugar stored in liver and skeletal muscle cells that is broken down to glucose and used by the body when it requires quick energy

glycosuria a condition characterized by the presence of glucose in the urine

gout a hereditary condition characterized by excessive amounts of uric acid (a product of protein breakdown) in the blood which crystallizes and is deposited in joints and in kidney tissue *guanine* one of the four purines that make up the genetic code in DNA

guarana seed a seed from the Brazilian shrub *Paullinia cupana* which is ground to a paste and ingested in a drink or in wafer bars for its high caffeine content

heroin a semisynthetic opiate produced by a chemical modification of morphine

hypertension a condition characterized by high blood pressure

hyperventilation excessive depth and rate of respiration leading to abnormal loss of carbon dioxide in the blood

hypokalemia a deficiency of potassium in the blood

infusion the steeping or soaking of a substance in order to extract its characteristic chemicals, such as caffeine from a tea leaf

ketonuria a condition seen in diabetics and characterized by reduced or disturbed carbohydrate metabolism

kola nut the bitter, caffeine-containing seed of the tree *Cola nitida* which is chewed or used in a drink

marijuana the leaves, flowers, buds, and/or branches of the hemp plant *Cannabis sativa* or *Cannabis indica* that contains cannabinoids, a group of intoxicating drugs

maté a South American holly, *Ilex paraguayensis,* whose caffeine-containing leaves and young shoots are used to make a drink also called maté

metabolism the chemical changes in the living cell by which energy is provided for the vital processes and activities and by which new material is assimilated to repair cell structure; or, the process that uses enzymes to convert one substance into compounds that can be easily eliminated from the body

methyl group CH_3; a molecule consisting of one carbon atom and three hydrogen atoms, usually found attached to other compounds

morphine the principal psychoactive ingredient of opium, which produces sleep or a state of stupor; the standard against which all morphine-like drugs are compared

mutagenesis the occurrence of mutations in a cell, often exhibited as cell character change and/or uncontrolled cell reproduction; caused by mutagens, or mutagenic agents, such as mustard gas and radiation of various wavelengths

opiate   a compound from the milky juice of the poppy plant *Papaver somniferum,* including opium, morphine, codeine, and their derivatives, such as heroin

paracetamol   N-acetylpara-amino-phenol, or APAP; a potent analgesic and antipyretic chemically similar to aspirin yet without anti-inflammatory action

parenteral administration   a form of drug ingestion whose route of administration bypasses the gastrointestinal tract and instead includes the lungs, skin, ear, or vagina

peristaltic action   successive muscular movements or contractions, such as those in the intestines that move ingested food onward

pharmacology   the study of drugs and their effects on living organisms

physical dependence   an adaption of the body to the presence of a drug, such that its absence produces withdrawal symptoms

placebo   a substance that is pharmacologically inactive and is used as a control in experiments measuring the effectiveness of another substance, or is administered in order to satisfy the psychological needs of patients

psychoactive   altering mood and/or behaviour

psychological dependence   a condition in which the drug user craves a drug to maintain a sense of well-being and feels discomfort when deprived of it

purine   the parent compound, $C_5H_4N_4$, of such compounds as adenine, guanine, xanthine, and trimethylxanthine, or caffeine

receptor site   specialized areas located on dendrites which, when bound by a specific number of neurotransmitter molecules, produce an electrical charge

REM sleep   rapid-eye-movement sleep; the phase of sleep, characterized by a specific type of electrical activity in the brain, during which dreaming takes place

solvent   a substance that is capable of dissolving one or more other substances; e.g., methylene chloride is the solvent used to extract caffeine from coffee beans

synergism   when two drugs together produce effects greater than either one could produce alone

synaptic gap   the space between the axon and the dendrite of two adjacent neurons in which neurotransmitters travel

tachycardia rapid heart or pulse rate

tea polyphenol oxidase an enzyme present in the sap of tea leaves that changes the flavour and colour of the leaves, thus producing black tea's characteristic taste and appearance; in green tea this chemical has been destroyed

theobromine a dimethylxanthine found in cocoa products, tea, and kola nuts whose effect on the body is similar, though only one-tenth as stimulating, as caffeine

theophylline a dimethylxanthine found in small amounts in tea whose stimulatory effect on the heart and breathing is stronger than caffeine; medically used in treating diseases in which breathing is difficult, such as asthma, bronchitis, and emphysema

thymine one of the four basic letters of the genetic code in the DNA molecule

tolerance a decrease of susceptibility to the effects of a drug due to its continued administration, resulting in the user's need to increase the drug dosage in order to achieve the effects experienced previously

toxic causing temporary or permanent damage to cells or organ systems of the body

tranquillizer a drug that has calming, relaxing effects

uric acid the main excreted substance produced by the breakdown of protein

ventricular fibrillation very rapid uncoordinated contractions of the ventricles of the heart resulting in a loss of synchronization of heartbeat and pulse

withdrawal the physiological and psychological effects of discontinued use of a drug

xanthine dioxypurine, $C_5H_4H_4O_2$; a purine that is an intermediate product of the liver's breakdown of the more complex purines to uric acid

yaupon cassina; the plant *Ilex cassine* or *Ilex vomitoria* whose caffeine-containing leaves and berries are used to make a tea

yoco bark the plant *Paullinia yoca* whose caffeine-containing bark is used to make a tea

Index

Richard Gilbert, Ph.D., has taught experimental psychology at universities in Scotland, Ireland, Canada, Mexico, and the United States. Since 1968 he has been associated with the Addiction Research Foundation of Ontario as a researcher and writer on the use and abuse of popular drugs, mostly alcohol, caffeine, and nicotine. He has written some 80 articles for scientific and scholarly journals.

Solomon H. Snyder, M.D., is Distinguished Service Professor of Neuroscience, Pharamacology and Psychiatry at The Johns Hopkins University School of Medicine. He has served as president of the Society for Neuroscience and in 1978 received the Albert Lasker Award in Medical Research. He is the author of *Uses of Marijuana, Madness and the Brain, The Troubled Mind, Biological Aspects of mental Disorder,* and edited *Perspective in Neuropharmacology: A Tribute to Julius Axelrod.* Professor Snyder was a research associate with Dr Axelrod at the National Institute of Health.

Malcolm Lader, D.Sc., Ph.D.,M.D., F.R.C. Psych. is Professor of Clinical Psychopharmacology at the Institute of Psychiatry, University of London and Honorary Consultant to the Bethlam Royal and Maudsley Hospitals. He is a member of the External Scientific Staff of the Medical Research Council. He has researched extensively into the actions of drugs used to treat psychiatric illness and symptoms, in particular the tranquillizers. He has written several books and over 300 scientific articles. Professor Lader is a member of several governmental advisory committees concerned with drugs.

Malcolm S. Bruce, M.R.C. Psych., is currently undertaking research into the effects of caffeine at the Institute of Psychiatry, London. His initial training in medicine was in Scotland, this was followed by specialization in psychiatry at St Thomas' Hospital, London. Since 1985 he has been in his present post as a Ph.D. student.